LETTING GO

Dr Charlie Corke (MB BS, BSc., MRCP[UK], FCICM) is one of Australia's leading Intensive Care specialists and is currently President of the College of Intensive Care of Australia and New Zealand. He is the regional clinical lead for the Advance Care Planning program and is the originator of the MyValues approach to advance care planning (myvalues.org.au). Dr Corke lectures widely on medical communication and end-of-life decision-making, was featured on the ABC in the film *In the End*, and is a regular contributor to radio.

Letting go

How to plan for a good death

Dr Charlie Corke

SCRIBE
Melbourne • London

Scribe Publications
18–20 Edward St, Brunswick, Victoria 3056, Australia
2 John St, Clerkenwell, London, WC1N 2ES, United Kingdom

Published by Scribe 2018

Typeset in 11.5/16.65 pt Adobe Garamond Pro by the publishers
Printed and bound in the UK by CPI Group (UK) Ltd, Croydon CR0 4YY

Scribe Publications is committed to the sustainable use of natural resources and
the use of paper products made responsibly from those resources.

9781911344858 (UK edition)
9781947534438 (US edition)
9781925322705 (Australian edition)
9781925548723 (e-book)

CiP data records for this title are available from the British Library and National
Library of Australia.

scribepublications.co.uk
scribepublications.com
scribepublications.com.au

This book is dedicated to all the amazing patients
and families who have travelled this path
with courage and compassion.

'Ours is a death-denying society and medicine
is a death-denying profession.'

—David Kuhl

'What tormented Ivan Ilyich most was the deception,
the lie, which for some reason they all accepted, that he
was not dying but was simply ill, and he only need keep
quiet and undergo treatment and something very good
would result.'

—Leo Tolstoy, *The Death of Ivan Ilyich*

'The waning days of our lives are given over to
treatments that addle our brains and sap our bodies
for a sliver's chance of benefit. These days are spent
in institutions — nursing homes and intensive care
units — where regimented, anonymous routines cut
us off from all the things that matter to us in life.'

—Atul Gawande

'Lives are like stories. The ending matters. Good stories
don't have bad endings. Our lives are a composition
of everything and the last bit matters just as much
as everything else.'

—Anon

Contents

Author's Note

This book is written from the context of an Australian doctor working in the Australian healthcare system. However, the dilemmas are universal. Experiences shared at international scientific meetings and those shared in discussions with colleagues from all over the world make it perfectly clear that the issues confronted in this book resonate everywhere.

Inevitably, there are subtle differences. The USA has a longer history of advance care planning than other countries. Most of this activity has been at a community level, with church social groups frequently playing a significant role. Planning is not specifically directed at those who are ill or in the last stages of life; instead, planning is advocated for those who are healthy. The general message relates to the writing of 'living wills', involving specific instruction about treatments that will be refused, rather than identifying outcomes that would be unacceptable or values that are important to the individual.

The landmark case of Karen Ann Quinlan in the 1970s (re Quinlan, 70 N.J. 10, 355 A.2d 647 (1976)) highlighted the importance of clearly declaring wishes regarding life-sustaining care. The court sought evidence that Karen had formally expressed her refusal of life-sustaining measures in the specific circumstances of her vegetative state. However, before the accident she had been a perfectly fit young woman and she hadn't expressed any opinion. The court was concerned that in the absence of a clear and specific refusal of life-sustaining measures, they had a duty to ensure that life-sustaining treatment be continued. In response to this case, living wills were advocated as a mechanism through which people could make clear those treatments that they would not want.

About the same time, durable powers of attorney for health care (or 'health care proxies') were introduced and quickly became law in every state. These individuals were empowered to make medical decisions for the person appointing them (with similar authority to the person who appointed them). In Australia, these people are called 'agents' or MEPOAs (Medical Enduring Powers of Attorney).

The benefits of advance care planning remained relatively uncontroversial in the USA until the introduction of the Patient Protection and Affordable Care Act ('Obama Care'), where Republicans suggested that any discussion about limiting intervention amounted to government-sponsored 'death panels'. This perception persists in some groups in the USA, but is not a widely held view elsewhere. Within the USA, African-Americans seem more likely than other racial groups to want lives prolonged as much as possible — even in cases of irreversible coma. Mistrust of doctors' predictions, faith in divine intervention, and a perception that the medical system discriminates against African-Americans appear to be major factors (the case of Jahi McMath is an illustration of this).

The requirement for 'living wills' to be highly specific, with a focus on refused treatments, has been recognised as somewhat unsatisfactory (either because people don't do them or because when they do, they turn out to be inadequate).

An alternative program, which involves doctors, has proved effective. Physician Orders for Life-Sustaining Treatment (POLST), also developed in the USA, helps ensure that a patient's wishes are followed. In this process, doctors, who know their patient's wishes, document these as a specific instruction. These letters combine the authority of a doctor's instruction with the authority of patient autonomy — i.e., doing what the patient wants — providing the reassurance that enables wishes to be respected. To be a valid POLST, though, depends on meaningful discussion of options and preferences between patients and clinicians, and this may not reliably occur.

In contrast to the privatised health system of the USA, UK health care is a national program (the National Health Service, or NHS). This provides a more uniform system of policies and procedures across the country that is more similar to that in Australia. Various policy documents advocate advance care planning including 'End of Life Care Strategy' (England and Wales), 'Living and Dying Well'

(Scotland), and 'Living Matters: Dying Matters' (Northern Ireland).

Advance care planning in the UK has more focus on the patient population, especially those with life-limiting illnesses. It tends to try to identify patient preferences rather than to elicit specific 'instructions' and doesn't talk of 'living wills'. The UK has a 'Preferred Priorities for Care' (PPC) document that is designed to facilitate communication between patients, health care providers, and family — rather than being a legal document (or 'instruction') in its own right. It provides information rather than instruction.

Appointment of a surrogate decision maker — called a Lasting Power of Attorney (LPA) in the UK — requires the involvement of a lawyer. This requirement may contribute to limited uptake, especially among those who are socially and financially disadvantaged, who are the least likely to do advance care planning

Despite differences in approach between regions, the challenges of advance care planning are similar — relatively few people plan for serious illness and even fewer document anything at all, leaving families and health care providers wondering exactly what the patient might want.

As a doctor, and an intensive-care specialist, I have looked after thousands of sick patients over many years. The vast majority survived, went home, and did well. These represent the good stories, the triumph of modern medicine, certainly the best part of my job. For these patients, decisions have generally been very straightforward, with little question that treatment was the 'right' thing to do or that the treatment was wanted.

But this book isn't about these great stories. It's about those for whom life is falling apart, whose pre-existing health and future prospects are bad, and where outcomes of treatment have become predictably poor or inadequate (in their judgment).

This book explores the choices we make in these situations, and how poor choices can make the last bit of life so much worse.

As we fade towards the end of our life, we will increasingly confront situations where it would be quite reasonable to 'let death happen', but where it is also possible (and perfectly reasonable) to try to 'do everything' to save or prolong life. It all depends on the wishes of the person who is sick.

These wishes are frequently unknown or unclear, but the decisions still have to be made.

Too frequently, we leave it until crisis strikes to start to think — but a crisis is never the best time for careful thought, especially about something difficult.

When stark choices have never before been considered, the need to decide comes as a huge shock to families as they gather anxiously in an unfamiliar waiting room. Few are prepared for the task and many find the process impossible, generally electing to do something because it is just too difficult to do nothing. Doctors find it no easier, and, without very clear instruction or permission to 'stand back', almost every doctor will strive to save life.

Saving, healing, and curing are core principles of medical practice: for doctors, letting someone die is fundamentally at odds with this medical imperative.

Most of us don't want to leave problems for our family — that's why we make a will. Planning for end-of-life decisions is just the same. Doing nothing risks causing distress and conflict for those left behind.

Death isn't something we can avoid. Assuming the natural order of things, our grandparents sicken and die, then our parents fail and die then, finally, it's us (along with others in our generation). At each step of this process, we are confronted with decisions about 'how far to go' and when to 'let go'. We keep being involved, initially as bystanders and finally as participants.

Medicine now makes it very easy to 'go too far', making it vital to set limits — unless, of course, you are one of those (few) who would 'never, never, want to give up' — for you, modern medicine has lots to offer, and generally delivers. But for those who have limits, it has become essential to communicate these.

As we struggle to make difficult decisions, it is important to be aware of things that might be influencing our decision-making. Recognising these influences helps us make wise decisions.

This book includes many stories that illustrate the numerous issues and dilemmas that can surround these difficult decisions.

These stories come from more than 20 years of medical

practice. All are based on real cases, though names and circumstances have been altered, as appropriate, to protect privacy. Some stories are a fusion of a number of similar episodes (to avoid repetition and convey clearer messages). Some are personal.

I thank all those who have taught me, and all those whose experiences have contributed to the stories in this book.

I hope it will encourage more thought, better decision-making, and clearer planning that will lead to more appropriate, compassionate care.

CHAPTER 1

We all have to go sometime

It had been a busy, but not particularly unusual, day. I was completing the evening ward round in the Intensive Care Unit (ICU) when I was called to see Judy.

The medical intern wanted Judy admitted to the ICU. She had come to the medical ward the night before with a serious pneumonia, and, despite powerful antibiotics, she was continuing to deteriorate.

I went down to see her. The intern was right to be worried. Judy sat bolt upright in bed, struggling to breathe. She was amazingly thin, with almost no muscle left. I estimated her to weigh little more than 35kg. She looked well beyond her 79 years.

With every breath her eyes bulged and her neck tightened, as she used every muscle in the failing effort to get air into her damaged lungs. Sweat glistened on her forehead. Her skin was an ominous grey. Her lips were blue.

A bedside monitor showed very little oxygen in her blood, and that her heart rate was much too slow for the effort she was making. It all suggested that her breathing or her heart would stop at any moment.

I held her hand. She gave no response.

Beside me, the intern recounted the medical history. Judy had serious lung disease that had relentlessly progressed, despite treatment.

Before this crisis, she could walk only a few yards, the least effort resulting in distressing breathlessness. A simple trip to the toilet had become a major undertaking.

Tests confirmed severe, end-stage lung disease.

Judy had been rejected for a lung transplant because of her age and her poor general condition. So that wasn't a possibility.

We needed to make a treatment decision, and quickly.

It wasn't an easy choice. With her severe lung disease, frail state, and advanced age, it was likely that nothing we could do would stop Judy from dying — but trying *would* risk drawing out her end unpleasantly (with needles, tubes, turning, and suctioning).

Alternatively, we could accept that Judy was dying. We could see this crisis as the final step in a progressive decline. We could give her enough medication to relieve any distress with her breathing; taking this course would mean that Judy would die quite quickly.

But we couldn't say, with absolute certainly, that Judy *couldn't* survive this acute illness. It wouldn't be *totally* futile to try — if that was what Judy wanted.

Were Judy to pull through (which was unlikely), it would take a long time and involve a big struggle on her part. Afterwards, she would be able to do even less than before she came to hospital (because serious illness in frail people almost always takes a toll). But it was possible that Judy would accept all this in order to live.

To save Judy (or to try, at least) would involve putting her on a breathing machine together with other intensive treatment. We certainly could do this — but should we?

To answer that question, we needed to know what Judy would want. We urgently needed to find out.

Judy was well beyond being able to tell us. There were no plans in place, even though this crisis was predictable. Like most people, Judy had never planned for this and her doctors had never raised it with her.

Henry, Judy's husband, was waiting anxiously. He didn't know what Judy would want. It was not something that they had ever discussed. He said that she wouldn't want to die, but that she wouldn't want to suffer. He wanted her to be 'given a chance'.

It was obvious that we had no permission to 'stand back' from attempting to save Judy, no permission to focus on comfort rather than cure. On the contrary, there was an expectation (from the medical team and from Henry) that we 'do everything' to try to save her.

We were still struggling to work out what to do when Judy stopped breathing.

Our hand was forced. We resuscitated her. We put a tube in her trachea and supported her with a mechanical ventilator. We took her to the ICU.

She went on to have a tracheostomy, and another tube inserted into her stomach through her nose so that we could feed her. Over the next weeks, she had numerous catheters inserted into the veins in her neck.

Repeatedly, she had to have tubes pushed in through her thin chest wall to drain the fluid that kept accumulating around her lungs. She needed repeated courses of antibiotics that caused profound diarrhoea, making her bottom very sore and excoriated. Despite the best of nursing care, her fragile skin broke down.

Eventually, the pneumonia resolved, sedation was reduced, and we tried to get Judy to breathe again for herself (as we turned down the mechanical support). This was an essential step if she was ever to be able to get off the ventilator — but it was always going to be difficult because Judy's lungs were dreadful.

These breathing trials went poorly. Each time the mechanical assistance was reduced, Judy quickly tired and her breathing failed.

Each time she failed, we put her back onto full breathing support.

Throughout her stay with us, Judy's communication was never clear, even after the sedation was reduced. She couldn't talk because the tracheostomy bypassed her vocal cords, and her writing was so shaky and jumbled that it was unreadable. Sedating drugs played a part in this, but without medication, her distress was obvious.

Judy resisted physiotherapy, and fought when blood was being taken, but it wasn't clear whether this represented a conscious refusal or was simply the result of delirium and confusion.

Eventually, Judy developed a chest infection that was profoundly antibiotic-resistant, at about the same time that her kidneys failed.

There was a conference of the entire medical team where it was agreed that Judy could not, and would not, survive.

Her family accepted this. They spent time with her, until she was taken off the mechanical ventilator on deep sedation (to ensure she would not experience the awful distress of being unable to breathe). It was agreed that, this time, we would not put her back on the ventilator when she failed.

Judy took only a few small breaths and that was that. She lay peacefully, as if asleep, her husband, Henry, holding her hand.

Afterwards, lying motionless, she seemed so small, so fragile, so violated. I felt we had let her down. We had been forced to, though, by the absence of any plan, or any limits. We had made her end worse than it could have been, and it was possible that we had given her exactly the sort of end that she really didn't want.

We will never know.

However much we try to avoid the prospect, or postpone the reality, we eventually die — all of us. We can't avoid it.

Humans have the unnerving capacity to anticipate our fate. Knowing should enable us to manage our end, but mostly we choose to ignore the opportunity and behave as if death is something we can avoid: something that happens to other people or something in the hands of a greater power.

In the past, medical treatment was so ineffective that it was rarely possible to do much to prevent death, so planning wasn't important. But things have changed. Effective life-support has become widely available over the last few decades (ICUs only started in the 1960s). With this, we have enormous power to artificially prolong life. Our medical progress makes dying very difficult.

It is not my intention in this book to malign modern medicine. I am a huge supporter; medical advances have brought tremendous benefit. Preventable, premature death has been almost entirely abolished, and this means that most of us can expect to live well into old age. It is a triumph.

Roy can attest to this.

Roy's story

An old neighbour of mine, Roy is a keen horse-trainer. He mostly trains his own horses, always hoping that the next will be 'that special one'.

One day, as he was riding, he blacked out and fell off. More accurately, Roy didn't fall but rolled off, doing himself no real damage in the process.

The horse was unfazed — Roy trains them to be

calm. Unfortunately, Roy had come off because he had become unconscious as a result of a cardiac arrest.

Roy's daughter started cardiopulmonary resuscitation (CPR), and his son-in-law called an ambulance. They were there in five minutes — they weren't far from town.

The crew shocked Roy back into a stable, effective heart rhythm and took him straight to hospital. A tight blockage in one of the main coronary arteries (supplying blood to his heart) was quickly identified, opened up, and a stent put in to keep it open. All this was done so quickly that the heart muscle beyond the blockage recovered nicely.

That evening, Roy watched the news while he ate his supper. He was discharged the next day and remains well.

Roy is still training and still hoping to find that special horse.

This is just one of many stunning stories. Stories where the threat of death or serious disability has been thwarted in a flash, by great systems, great expertise, and great technology. These are now everyday stories, the fantastic legacy of modern medicine.

The inevitable effect of preventing premature death, though, is that we will be that much older when we die (or have our final illness). And advanced age comes with progressive decline and debility that medicine may relieve but can't reverse.

Our ability to keep on treating — as well as the fact that treatment needs to become more intensive as we decline and become sicker, complications get more common, and recovery more unlikely and more difficult — makes it important for us to consider how far we want to go.

'How far' is something very personal, a question that we all answer differently. Some want to hold on to life with fingernails, 'never to give in', to value every living moment, to 'try, try, and try again'. These people are willing to accept whatever burden is required to stay alive. They contend that 'life wasn't meant to be easy' and believe that suffering is an integral part of life. I had a great uncle who expressed exactly this sort of attitude.

Others take a very different approach. They prefer to get out early, to avoid as much badness as possible, to go without fuss. They want 'out' as soon as the quality of life drops, dignity is compromised, or independence is lost. In their view, pain and suffering are negative and pointless. They see no glory in fighting a losing battle, or in the battle itself. My mother-in-law was like this.

Doing our best to keep people alive is almost instinctive — both as doctors and as people. It seems so right. We do it for the best of reasons. But it can have unfortunate consequences. There is always one case that stands out. Over my career, I have been honoured with invitations to teach overseas, and during these visits I am often invited to participate in medical rounds to discuss the management of patients. It was during a visit to China that I encountered Mrs Li.

Mrs Li's story

From the very start of the round, there was an air of excitement. They would be showing me 'a special patient'. There was an expectation that I would be impressed.

Anticipation mounted as we went from patient to patient. Finally, we arrived at the room of Mrs Li, the 'special patient'. (I never heard anyone use a first name, so I, too, will call her 'Mrs Li'.)

One of the junior doctors presented the case. He explained how Mrs Li had come to the hospital 10 years earlier. At that time, she had been unable to breathe as a result of advanced motor neurone disease. This decline in her breathing had relentlessly progressed over the preceding two years — a story that sounded pretty much typical for the classic, aggressive version of the disease.[1]

The Chinese team wanted me to appreciate a triumph of their medical practice and nursing care — and I was certainly impressed with their ability. They had kept Mrs Li going for 10 years in a state of total paralysis. They had avoided overwhelming pneumonia, avoided losing her to a serious urinary infection, prevented lethal clot

---

1 Motor neurone disease (MND) is a terrible condition characterised by progressive loss of muscle power that causes a relentlessly increasing paralysis. Characteristically, the ability to breathe and swallow is lost within two years (with the ability to move limbs being lost well before this). Cruelly, consciousness and sensation remain completely unaffected. When breathing eventually fails, artificial mechanical ventilation can extend survival, but usually by only a few months. Mechanical ventilation requires the creation of a tracheostomy and this usually means that any remaining ability to speak or swallow will be lost. This makes communication very difficult because the ability to write or type will typically have been lost long before. When the ability to breathe is lost, many people conclude that mechanical ventilation is not a good idea because ongoing life (without the ability to move, breathe or communicate effectively) is not 'worth it'. Dying becomes preferable.

formation, prevented bedsores — it was amazing. I had never before seen anyone so debilitated survive without complication for so long.

But it felt totally wrong; it seemed to be excellence without reason. Nobody seemed to have considered Mrs Li's best interests. There seemed no concern for how she might have suffered (or could still be suffering).

Respectfully, I enquired about Mrs Li's wishes. I wanted to know if this outcome was something that Mrs Li might have wanted (though I couldn't personally imagine that anyone would want this). I wanted to understand what the team felt they were achieving for her. They didn't appear to understand my question — they had done so well, why would I question them?

It seemed that during her first year on mechanical ventilation, Mrs Li had progressively lost all ability to communicate. During that time, there had been no discussion with Mrs Li about her wishes.

Mrs Li's family was relatively wealthy. They regularly paid the modest fee that the hospital required. They had retained Mrs Li's long-time 'amah' (maid), Zhou, to look after her in the hospital. Every day Zhou came in, changed Mrs Li's nappy, tenderly washed her, and sang to her. She combed Mrs Li's long hair and carefully applied her make- up. All day I saw Zhou busily attending to Mrs Li as she lay there, immaculate and unresponsive. Always in freshly laundered, beautifully embroidered silk pyjamas.

On examination, Mrs Li had large, fixed, and dilated pupils. This is a grave sign that the connection between the light reaching the eye and the nerve controlling the contraction of the pupil is broken (usually due to profound brain damage). It's a very basic reflex, so its absence was telling. I checked for other brain reflexes, but found none. This was evidence that Mrs Li's brain was not functioning, even at the most rudimentary level. It meant that she was totally unconscious and unaware. In the circumstances, I felt relieved by this — it suggested that she could not be suffering. However, it was impossible to know for how long, or how much, Mrs Li might have suffered before unconsciousness supervened. This was disturbing — it could have been years.

The doctors and nurses treating Mrs Li weren't unkind — not at all. They were kind, intelligent, and very dedicated. I think they would have been upset if they thought that they might have been responsible for causing terrible distress to Mrs Li. Nor do I doubt that Mrs Li's family loved her very much, and believed that they were doing their best.

Zhou's dedication was likewise obvious.

Unfortunately, the determination of everyone to 'do the very best', without thinking of the consequences, provided a stark example of where all this can lead.

As we focus on the *disease* it is very easy to forget the *person* behind the disease. This concept isn't new, but it seems we need constant reminding. William Osler, a leading physician in Victorian times, observed that, 'It is more important to know what sort of a patient has a disease than what sort of a disease a patient has.' His advice is even more pertinent today.

Some years ago, we ran focus groups to help us to understand how people think about medical treatment towards the end of life. We brought together a fabulous group of elderly ladies who were all volunteers in a large nursing home. All were over 75 years old. They were funny, frank, and insightful.

One started with the classic statement: 'I'm not worried, because when the time comes my doctor and family will know what to do.' By this, she meant they would know when to stand back and 'let her go'.

The others disagreed. They didn't think their family would have the confidence to stop. Some shared stories of times they believed doctors and families had gone 'much too far'.

In the end, they all agreed that they needed to clearly instruct their families about what would be 'too far', and tell them what they were keen to avoid. None thought that their family would have sufficient confidence to hold back without being specifically told to do so. They all agreed that their families would need to be given 'permission not to push'.

One woman suggested that if a condition could be treated, there was an obligation to try. This resulted in general agreement that simple treatments (such as antibiotics) should generally be accepted, but other 'excessive' and 'burdensome' treatments (like long-term mechanical ventilation or dialysis) could reasonably be declined. They observed that a treatment that might be regarded as excessively burdensome by one person might be considered to be acceptable by somebody else.

They went on to talk about 'toughness', and how some people seem willing to tolerate a great deal of 'badness' (by which they meant burdensome treatment with poor outcomes) in order to live. Interestingly, all of them recoiled from the possibility of much 'badness' for themselves. They felt that there could be no hard and fast rules about 'how far to go', agreeing that this would be very difficult, if not impossible, to predict for another person.

All of them valued the availability of medical treatment. They recognised that most of them 'wouldn't be here now' without modern medicine. They were right. Between them, they had pacemakers, artificial hips, knee replacements, coronary bypasses, and heart valves. All were taking medication of some sort, most were on lots of tablets, and two were on insulin ... they were a vibrant example of the benefit of modern medicine!

But they nonetheless recognised that medicine had limits.

None of them were looking forward to dying, and none

of them were ready to die. But all were prepared for the possibility and, indeed, the inevitability of death. They just hoped that theirs wouldn't be too bad. They wanted it to be uncomplicated and quick.

They all recognised that medical treatment had the potential to make their end more difficult and unpleasant.

Their comments were revealing. Years later, I still reflect on how this lovely group summed up all the complexities of end-of-life treatment decision-making — far better than most forums of medical experts.

However, it was striking that, despite their clarity of thought, *not one* of them had completed any sort of written plan to record their wishes, and none felt that they had had a proper conversation with their family about their wishes! Other focus groups, involving younger participants, found the topic much more difficult to discuss. They readily identified situations that they considered intolerable (almost everyone can think of some), but were unwilling to forgo treatments — even treatment that would achieve an outcome they had already identified as being unacceptable. They held to the idea that there could be a surprise, good outcome — that miracle that we all hope for. For these younger groups, hope, even completely unrealistic hope, prevented them setting down a clear 'line in the sand', when they would want others to step back and let them die. Inevitably, there were exceptions, but these were uncommon. The ambivalence of these younger participants should not distract from the clarity of thought we saw among the older group, though, for whom severe illness and death were more real and proximate.

Hope (even unrealistic hope) can be an important driver that keeps us going. It is human to hope, especially when we are confronted by something terrible, like dying.

We hope for the impossible; we make a virtue of it.

But hope has a price. The philosopher Friedrich Nietzsche took a dim view of it, writing: 'Hope, in reality, is the worst of all evils because it prolongs the torments of man.' His take is reflected in the mythological story of Pandora. We are told that Pandora possessed a box that constrained all the terrors and torments of humanity. When she unwisely opened the box, she unleashed all these to wreak havoc on the world. Realising her error, Pandora quickly reclosed the box, trapping 'hope' inside. The story suggests that hope was not in the box by accident — it was there because its potential to torment was recognised long ago.

Dealing with hope is difficult. It is common, and natural, to hold on to hope when treatments fail and grim death looms. But blind hope means never, ever giving up, never stepping back, and forever escalating the intensity of treatment. This can easily lead to a lot of burdensome, futile technology before death finally comes, and a process of dying that many would consider to be 'bad'.

We commonly assume that hope means rejecting reality ('We are still clinging on to hope so we don't want to think about that.') However, it is important to recognise that it can be perfectly possible and reasonable to be hopeful and realistic at the same time: to 'hope for the best and plan for the rest', as one family put it to me. There is no harm in hanging on to hope, providing we ensure that we don't let it block reasonable, compassionate decisions (or decisions the person themselves would want).

Doctors and family feel a tremendous responsibility to 'do something' to save (or extend) life. This happens however unpleasant and prolonged the medical journey is likely to be — and however poor the outcome.

By the time everyone comes to agree that treatment can *never* work, the patient will have gone through an awful lot.

When we think rationally (or indeed, when we start to think about it at all), most of us have concerns about how bad our end might be, and share a desire to mitigate this. Most of us can imagine situations where we believe we would prefer to be dead than to endure. Few of us want our lives extended indefinitely 'at any cost'.

The human hope to vanquish death is not new. Over ages, death has been seen as an exquisite evil. Artists have dramatically portrayed death as the black-robed, skeletal reaper — an image that chills us. Collectively, we think of death as so awful that we have to avoid it.

Contrasting ideas portray death as a release from suffering, a 'rest in peace', recognising that for everyone, at some time, 'it's OK to die'. In this view, death is portrayed as a relief. It recognises a courageous grace in acceptance.

Balancing these different ideas proves very difficult for patients, families, doctors, nurses — everyone.

Saving becomes an easy default, and treatment progressively escalates until even the most optimistic (delusional or unrealistic) family member or doctor finally comes to accept that death is unavoidable. This can take a long time and involve a lot of intervention.

Recognising all this, we might consider the circumstances that are likely to surround our own death (in a developed Western society):

Most of us who live in developed countries will die, after a long period of declining health and function, sometime in our eighth decade — and not as a result of a sudden final illness striking while we are otherwise well.

Someone will call an ambulance, and this will take us to hospital. We will be unconscious (or too sick to reliably say what we want). We won't have a plan or wishes documented (because few do).

Our family will be unable to confidently agree about our wishes for medical treatment ('how far' we would want to go). In the absence of certainty or consensus to stand back, medical intervention will escalate.

We will spend our last days connected to machines, cared for by strangers, and separated from our family.

We will experience significant suffering, discomfort, and indignity, receiving increasingly intense treatment that has a diminishing chance of success.

Medical technology will dominate our last days and weeks. Our family will be excluded from the bedside, huddled in the waiting room, while 'important' things are done to us. Time for connection and comforting, for any sort of intimacy or the opportunity to say goodbyes, will be missed (or compromised).

It's a worrying prospect.

Most chronically sick, elderly people do not seek, and may actively fear, the prospect of intensive medical technology at the end of life. For many, the 'fear of death' has been replaced by the 'fear of dying'.

Today, life-support treatment is eventually limited or discontinued in up to 70 per cent of patients who die in Intensive Care Units in Australia. Rates of discontinuation are generally somewhat lower elsewhere, but, clearly, a lot of intensive treatment is being provided that does not (and cannot) work.

There are substantial regional differences. The incidence of withdrawal of life-sustaining treatments ranges from 48 per cent in northern Europe to just 18 per cent in the south. Some suggest that this can be explained by the tendency of Catholic medical staff in southern Europe (as opposed to Protestants and agnostics in the north) to be less likely to withdraw treatment. The same may apply to families.

In the latter stages of life, there may well come a time when celebrating the fullness of a life already lived and knowing when it's time to go may be preferable to seeking to indefinitely extend a declining existence with relentless escalation of medical intervention.

Literature is an important way in which we convey sensitive concepts. Surely the most famous poem that embraces our approach to end of life must be 'Do not go gentle into that good night' by Dylan Thomas.

Thomas wrote his poem in reaction to his elderly father's progressive decline. His father had been a robust, strong man throughout his life, but in his old age became blind and weak. He was clearly failing at the time the poem was written. Thomas was disturbed to see his father become 'soft' and 'gentle', losing his 'spark' and 'fight'. No longer the 'fierce' man he had previously been. Thomas makes a passionate appeal to his father to fight, rather than to accept his fate.

It seems Thomas accurately reflected the common attitude of families as elderly parents deteriorate and die — an attitude I have seen so many times in my work.

Knowing when to let death 'have its way' has always been confronting and has become more difficult with advances in modern medicine. Doctors and family find stepping back from life-saving treatment virtually impossible, unless they have clear and determined instruction that this is the 'right' thing to do: that it is what the patient wants.

Most of these life-and-death decisions get made when the person concerned is beyond being able to make decisions (due to unconsciousness, delirium, or dementia) so decisions increasingly fall to doctors and families, who are often not at all confident about what the sick person would want.

These can feel like near impossible choices — and getting

it wrong is really, really serious. To 'let someone die' who would want to live is clearly inexcusable; and yet, to impose invasive, potentially degrading, treatment on someone who does not want it is equally unforgivable.

Throughout my career, I have witnessed many, many families agonising over treatment choices for a frail, elderly, dying relative. I am always struck by how much stress this causes when they don't know 'for sure' what their sick relative would want. It strikes me how few have had any meaningful discussion, even where deterioration has been progressing over many years.

While we do learn from others, it is often our own personal experience that has the most impact. I, too, have struggled in my role as family member.

Freddy's story

Freddy was my father. He was a man of his time — reserved and very proper. He found emotion difficult. He wasn't fun, but he was a good reliable parent, and the only one we had.

Our mother left us when my brother and I were very young. Her departure followed a sequence of flamboyant affairs that she had flaunted. It caused a huge scandal in the conservative atmosphere of the 1950s.

It must have been devastating for Dad, and I presume she must have been very mixed up.

She never returned or made any contact with us.

She simply disappeared. We were so young that we can't remember anything about her.

Dad only showed us a picture of her when he became a bit reflective in advanced old age. Throughout our lives, she was a forbidden topic of conversation, and we never asked. At that time, a 'clean break' was thought best.

After we'd both left home, Dad married Dot. She was wonderful, providing the happy, reliable, loving stability that he so needed.

Dad enjoyed good health, took no medication, and never had to go into hospital for anything. He managed his building company until he was over 80, and drove on local roads (a bit scarily!) till he was 86.

But good health can never last forever.

Shortly after his 90th birthday, his failing memory and frailty became unmistakable. Dot tried her best, but she couldn't cope. Eventually, Dad had to go into a nursing home. By then he was only saying a few words.

He deteriorated rapidly. Soon he was saying nothing, recognising nobody, and doing nothing for himself. He needed a hoist to move him from his bed to the chair.

Dot visited every day. She complimented the nursing staff and constantly reassured everyone of how well Dad was being cared for.

His eating became slower and increasingly difficult. His food was going down into his lungs. This caused continual bouts of pneumonia. Each was treated with a course of antibiotics.

Dot was concerned about Dad's deterioration. She wanted 'something done' to 'help him'. She had no clear idea what this something was, but he was given more potent antibiotic to allay her concern.

My brother and I were concerned that Dad had got into a situation that he would never have wanted. Throughout his life, he had regularly delivered a harsh assessment of nursing homes, describing them as 'pointless and degrading' places, where people 'exist waiting to die'. This might not have been an overly generous assessment, but it had been his unfailing view. He had left no doubt that he didn't want this for himself. Towards the end, he'd told me that he 'knew death was the next big thing ahead of him' and that he just wanted to 'get it over with as quickly as possible'.

We shared our concern with the GP. He said that he considered the antibiotic to be a simple treatment, one that would impose no particular burden on Dad. He explained that, in his opinion, only 'burdensome' treatments might reasonably be withheld. He felt that not giving antibiotics would be to intend to bring forward Dad's death, something he could never sanction. But he reassured us that Dad would die soon anyway, and he didn't think the antibiotic would make much difference. He also pointed out that Dot, as next of kin, wanted everything done to save Dad (he was certainly right about that) and that he was following her wishes.

Now things were complicated. To push Dad's wishes

would risk upsetting Dot and the GP. Dot was clearly devoted to Dad, and she was the nearest relative. The GP was acting in accordance with her instruction. My brother and I were peripheral.

Dot continued to focus on the hope that she wouldn't lose him. She avidly identified each new problem as soon as it developed and each time she pushed for treatment. For her, getting medical attention was simply a logical continuation of how she had cared for him all along.

It was impossible to advocate to 'stand back' without causing upset — and we didn't. The antibiotic worked and the pneumonia settled. Dad survived several more months. Dot visited him every day. He never showed any sign that he knew her.

I'm sure Dad wouldn't have felt that any of it was a good idea. But equally, he would never have wanted to upset Dot, and he wouldn't have wanted us to upset her either. It was all probably inevitable.

At least Dad couldn't tell the nurses how he felt about nursing homes.

Mabel's story

Mabel was my grandmother. Without our mum, school holidays were difficult for Dad, and each holiday my brother and I were sent on the train to stay with Mabel in London. We had a great time. She loved us utterly, and we looked forward to our trips.

My grandfather had been killed in the final days of the First World War, while Mabel was pregnant with my father. He was her fourth child. When he was born, Mabel had four children under five. She never remarried, never drank, never smoked, and worked tirelessly. To us, she was a perfect matriarch, always dependable and unfailingly supportive.

I never considered that she might get sick; she simply wasn't that sort of person. As she got older, she regularly visited much younger friends who were ill, describing them as 'poor old things'. Repeatedly, she asked us to promise that we would 'never ever let it happen' to her. This request encompassed a variety of bad outcomes including dementia, ending up in a nursing home, wearing a nappy ... the list was long, but the message was clear.

Eventually, as she approached her 90th birthday, her mental and physical heath started to fail. At first, there were subtle changes. She tried to cover these up, but the signs were there. She crocheted incessantly, and her deterioration was sadly documented in the increasing disarray in her blankets.

She continued to live at home, mostly because of the care she received from Aunt Margery (youngest of the three daughters). Margery had never married. She had been popular and she'd had boyfriends, but she saw her duty at home. In the straightforward way that children see these things, we appreciated having a fabulous auntie who spoiled us. She was a teacher who adored her children; she would have made a wonderful mother. Only much later did I come to appreciate the enormous sacrifice she had made.

Over the years, Mabel suffered lots of small, but potentially serious, medical problems. On each occasion, we all ensured that she got the best medical care as quickly as possible. As a medical student at the time, and the only medical member of our family, I was an enthusiastic participant.

As a result of our efforts, she survived a number of crises, while her dementia progressed, taking her to a state that she would have despised — that very situation we had promised 'never to let happen'. We didn't recognise what we were doing, of course, but everything we did ensured that it did happen.

At 92, she was incontinent and completely confused.

One morning, Aunt Margery found her in terrible distress. Her right leg was white and very cold. Subsequent, frantic family conversations concluded that she needed to be urgently sent to hospital. The GP was called as the first step — he had seen Mabel regularly and knew her. He came straight round (home visiting by GPs was remarkable in those days).

He instantly diagnosed the problem: a blood clot was totally blocking the arterial circulation to Mabel's leg. He discussed options.

He first explained that this event would almost

certainly prove fatal, whatever was done. He wondered if it might be better to keep Mabel at home, and reassured us that, if she stayed, he would ensure she had no pain.

As soon as we had absorbed this suggestion, it seemed perfectly obvious that it was the right thing to do: we knew she wanted to be at home at the end, and we knew that her current state was way, way beyond where she had ever wanted to be. We could see that trying to save her was the last thing she would have wanted us to do.

Our instinctive reaction to get her to hospital evaporated.

I'm sure this wise old doctor didn't notice the awkward medical student in the background, but I certainly remember him. He taught me something that I have never forgotten — the importance of providing confidence, common sense, and supportive guidance amidst the emotion of a medical crisis.

He gave decent pain relief, which worked wonders. Mabel remained completely settled and died peacefully a few hours later. We sat on the bed with her and talked till morning.

Looking back, I deeply regret how much we let her down. She would have been so upset to have seen herself in her last years. We'd promised her that we wouldn't let it happen, but we did.

We treated everything, and even at the very end we

wanted to do more. We did what many families do because we never thought to let go.

Much of the problem may come from our ability to deny the reality of death, and we have devised a number of ingenious ways to do this.

Only thinking of deterioration in terms of illness excludes thinking about dying. Illness requires treatment, and failed treatment signifies the need for more intense treatment. And so it goes on, until we are certain that nothing can work. 'Trying everything' in this way easily ends up in weeks or months of increasingly burdensome treatment, with all the suffering this may entail.

Thinking of (our) death and terminal illness as both something that we know that we *should* plan for, but also as something that is so very far into the future that it doesn't merit our attention 'just now', means that we don't *need* to think about it. We wait to 'cross that bridge when we come to it'. We can easily keep on with this 'not quite yet' attitude until it is far too late to plan at all.

The ready availability of advanced life support has made death 'optional' to the extent that it is now often necessary to make a clear (but difficult) decision to 'let it happen'.

Effective life support has only existed for the last few decades. This change has happened during my medical career, and I have found the speed of this change rather staggering.

When I qualified in 1977, the ward on which I worked was laid out in the traditional Nightingale design, with white painted metal beds all lined up in long rows, just the same as a century before.

The neatness of the bed making, with folded hospital corners in the sheets, was the measure of good nursing; patient outcomes didn't seem to come into it.

Medical practice depended, almost entirely, on the expert knowledge of the treating doctor. I can recall no protocols or guidelines being available to us at that time, and we certainly used none. We asked more senior doctors for advice, who sometimes knew and sometimes guessed.

We did our best, but it wasn't that good.

Though I was at the lowest part of the system, I felt responsible for poor outcomes, and I still do. To this day, I can recall many of those who died. People who certainly should not have died and who would not have died today. Adherence to appropriate and effective guidelines, timely escalation where things don't improve, highly skilled care, senior supervision, and effective medical treatments have now made things so much better.

Over the last few decades, ambulance services have developed, too, delivering highly effective life-saving treatment to virtually every street and every home. The same efficiency continues in modern emergency departments. Capabilities, organisation, and resources bear little resemblance to the service that existed when I graduated.

Hospital treatments have also evolved to an amazing extent. When I first worked as a doctor in 1977 (at a leading British hospital), patients who suffered a heart attack were treated with prolonged bed rest and then sent home. That was it. No clot busting, no stenting of blocked arteries, no heart surgery (with very rare exceptions). Results were predictably poor. Death within a year, from second or third attacks, was quite common.

Today, cardiac intervention is routine, rapid, and awesomely effective. Coronary artery disease is often diagnosed and treated within the same day, returning people to live productive, healthy lives. This is but one example, and there are many others.

We so readily adapt and accept new medical advances that we need reminding how far we have come. Today, we take the availability of life support for granted.

While we adopt advances quickly, we are slower to recognise their downside.

Now, for the first time, it is possible that medical treatment will prolong life longer than we might want, in a condition that we wouldn't accept. This has become a challenge for health care, for society, for families, and, most importantly, for every one of us as individuals.

Kerry's story

Kerry Packer, one of Australia's wealthiest men, suffered severe cardiac disease together with recurrent chronic renal failure at the end of his life.

Kerry had made headlines (and caused some controversy) some years earlier when his long-serving personal-helicopter pilot 'voluntarily' donated one of his kidneys to Kerry for transplantation.

Five years on, aged 68, Kerry's general health was poor and his transplanted kidney was failing.

The stage was reached where going back on dialysis was required to keep Kerry alive. This would have been relatively simple to perform and not especially burdensome in itself.

Kerry did not want his life prolonged with dialysis. He had had dialysis before, knew what was involved, and did not want it.

He told his cardiologist that he was 'running out of petrol' and wanted to 'die with dignity'. His wish was respected, and he died peacefully with his family in attendance.

Clearly, this was not a decision he made because of resource limitation. Kerry had enough money to obtain any medical treatment he desired, and he had previously done so. It was a decision based on his personal assessment of the burden of dialysis treatment and illness in relation to the benefit he perceived he would get from it.

CHAPTER 2

Why everyone feels they

have to save you

Though we might hope to have our wishes respected, it seems that we aren't really free to choose what we want to happen at the end of our lives. Almost everything and everyone is there to ensure that we are 'saved'. Many people, and institutions, feel that they have a right to be involved in this decision, and often have strong opinions.

Let's consider some of these influences.

Families generally believe that they have the right and the responsibility to make end-of-life decisions. They can be quite strident about this.

Society recognises the role of families. There is a widespread belief that the family has the right to decide to withdraw life support from a persistently comatose patient or unconscious patient (or to refuse to allow this to happen).

News stories regularly tell us that 'the family made the difficult decision to withdraw life support' — so it seems that the media think that it is the family's decision. Doctors routinely look to the patient's family when treatment decisions need to be made and the patient themselves can't make them, so they clearly think the family play a role, too.

Protection, love, and duty are strong instincts for family members, and these easily translate into advocacy to save the life of a beloved relative. Appeals to scientific reason or suggestions that the wishes of the sick relative be respected often prove ineffective in the face of such strong emotional instinct.

Let me share some examples of how this works.

Mark's story

Maggie kept her husband, Mark, at home as long as she could manage. She knew that he wanted to stay at home until the end, and she did her best. After 40 years of marriage, she felt it was the least she could do.

As Mark's dementia progressed, he became very dependent and increasingly difficult. Maggie couldn't cope. She made sure that she found the best nursing home for him.

She visited every day, ensuring that Mark was clean and dry, that his hair was brushed, and that he was eating. The standard she applied to everyday details seamlessly extended to his illnesses. The 'best' was to cure, to save, and to get him the best treatment. She had to do her best.

Whenever Mark was unwell, Maggie got the nurses to call the doctor immediately. She ensured that he attended quickly, and made sure that the medications he prescribed were given regularly and on time.

When Mark got very sick, Maggie made sure he was sent to the best private hospital to be seen by the best specialist.

Mark's dementia progressed to the stage where he stopped speaking and was no longer able to recognise Maggie (or anyone else). His swallowing became so bad that he was unable to stop food and drink from going into his lungs. His cough was so weak that he couldn't clear the inhaled food from his lungs. Inevitably, he developed a severe pneumonia. Despite antibiotics, he got worse. He was transferred to hospital where, inevitably, Maggie wanted 'everything' done.

Mark's breathing was failing. The next step would be to support his breathing with a breathing machine. This needed to be done in the Intensive Care Unit, so we were called in.

I asked Maggie to tell me about Mark. I got her to start by telling me how they had met ... after that, I said nothing (except to encourage Maggie to go on) for the next 15 minutes.

She told me how Mark had been a funny, dignified, determined man. She explained that their life had been good, with the inevitable challenges. Her story finished on that day in the emergency department. Telling the story helped Maggie to appreciate the gravity of the situation, in her own words.

I asked how she felt Mark would feel about his situation. She had no difficulty — Mark would be horrified. She said it would be the 'last thing he would have wanted' and something that he 'would never have accepted'. I asked what Mark would want us to do now. She said that he would tell us to 'let him go' — actually, she went further and used the words 'set him free'.

She cried.

I acknowledged how difficult this must be for her (I was concerned that she would feel that she was abandoning Mark). I made a point of admiring her dedication to him and acknowledging that I saw how much she loved him.

I reassured her we would make the decision together — Mark, Maggie, and I. Mark could contribute to the decision as his old self, a vibrant, funny, guy who didn't hesitate to say what he felt.

We agreed that it was time to stop.

Mark died peacefully with Maggie by his side, doing her best as always.

For some families, it is more about 'duty' than love or emotion. Duty can be very powerful, and this is often expressed as a grown child's responsibility to keep elderly parents alive.

Such duty can be very obvious in Chinese or Indian families, but it happens across cultures. 'Duty' makes the wishes of the parent almost irrelevant, so much so that they may not be considered at all.

Love can also be a potent motivation to 'save'. The influence of love and loveliness can't be understated. The illustrator Ronald Searle conveyed this beautifully. When his wife faced a serious illness, he created a series of beautiful pictures, depicting her as a delightful mole, in lovely settings.

These pictures were later gathered together as a small, whimsical book entitled *Les Très Riches Heures de Mrs Mole* (The Very Rich Hours of Mrs Mole).

In his own words, he described what he was intending:

'Everything about these (pictures) had to be romantic and perfect. I drew them originally for no one's eyes except Mo's, so she would look at them propped up against her bedside lamp and think: "When I'm better, everything will be beautiful."'

This was no pragmatic response to illness. This was a beautiful, and very personal, expression of love and hope. She was going to get better and everything would be beautiful.

Love and hope trump all else. They provide a tremendous drive to try to save. For many families, acceptance and letting go seem to be in direct contravention of love. It seems like love needs to be abandoned in order to let go — something impossible for those who *really* love.

The 'imperative of possibility' and the 'duty to save' are additional motivators to action. The power of possibility makes trying seem the right thing to do whenever a treatment *could* work (however unlikely this is and whatever the consequences of failure).

The obligation to save is so powerful that it makes attempting to save seem mandatory. It feels like a duty.

Because it is always possible to 'do something' (even where there is no chance of this working), we feel obligated to do it. This imperative drives us to 'do everything', to 'try', and encourages us to treat because we can. It's a powerful urge.

We feel obliged to provide something if it is available (this is the 'imperative of availability').

Let me give you an example that incorporates a number of these concepts. Imagine that someone arrives in hospital with a terrible injury. An injury that is so severe that, right from the start, it is quite obvious that it is not survivable. The appropriate action would be to do no advanced investigation and provide no invasive treatment.

In reality, however, scans will be done. These scans are readily available, quick, and easy in most big hospitals, and the more severe the injury, the more urgent the investigation becomes. The imperatives of possibility and availability make it seem unreasonable *not* to do the scan.

So ... a scan gets done and shows a large bleed inside the skull that is causing a severe compression of the brain (this would not be a surprise in a terrible injury).

Bleeds like this can be drained by surgery, and such operations are routine for neurosurgeons. Once again, it seems 'important' and 'right' that the blood is drained urgently.

From a rational perspective, it's illogical because it can't change the outcome, but it is easy to see why, in a crisis, 'doing something' seems so much better than 'doing nothing'. It explains how modern medicine, with so much possibility to 'do something', leads us to do so much.

Efficient systems also contribute to how much we do. The ready availability of investigation, tests, and intervention makes it so easy to start, and easy to move to the next step. It all feels so natural and so inevitable.

Margaret's story

Margaret was 89. She had severe dementia and could no longer recognise her family. They had managed her at home as long as they could, but she had been in a nursing home for the last year.

One day, the nurse rang Margaret's daughter, Susan, to say that Margaret was very unwell. The doctor had been informed and an ambulance had been called.

Soon after Margaret arrived in the emergency department, a major abdominal perforation was diagnosed. The local surgeon felt that Margaret was too sick for an operation in the small regional hospital, as he did not have ICU backup. Urgent transfer was arranged to our hospital.

Margaret got there first, while Susan was still driving in. The surgical registrar rang her on her mobile to ask her to 'give consent' for Margaret to have an operation. Susan gave consent; it seemed the expected thing to do.

A large, perforated gastric ulcer was found and repaired. After the operation, Margaret was so ill that she couldn't manage without mechanical ventilation (as the first surgeon had predicted) so she was transferred straight from the operating theatre to the ICU.

When Susan arrived, she was shocked. She realised that what had happened was not at all what Margaret would have wanted. She was sure that Margaret would not have wanted any 'heroics' (as she put it). The rest of the family felt the same.

Now Margaret was on life support in intensive care. The surgeon objected to stopping straight after he had just spent hours operating. He told the family that now the operation was done, things had to take their (medical) course.

Margaret eventually left ICU, but she didn't thrive, and died six weeks later without leaving hospital.

Lack of availability of services (or confident decision-making) often leads to transfer to a larger hospital, often over huge distances. The absence of technological capability frequently dominates the whole thought process, while a more balanced discussion of what would be best for Margaret, and what she would want, may well have been more appropriate.

The surgeon who operated on Margaret would be fairly typical, thinking that he had an agreement with Susan when she gave consent for 'everything' that was required to get Margaret through after the operation. This attitude can be a problem when patients and families decide to try heroic surgery, with the expectation that they will be able to bail out if it doesn't go as well as they hope. It can be confronting to find that they are locked in by the surgeon's view that what comes after is a necessary part of the process — including all the predicted, and often inevitable, complications.

This approach of 'whatever it takes' has been described as a 'covenantal' ethic. A 'covenant' involves a special sort of firm or sacred agreement and obligation. The surgeon makes a covenant with their patient when they promise to use their surgical skill to battle death on behalf of the patient. In return, the patient puts their trust in the surgeon and accepts whatever is required.

Once made, this contract makes it difficult (or impossible) for the patient to set limits or to bail out. Some surgeons refuse to operate *without* having an assurance that the patient will 'go the distance'.

One surgeon (well known for the ferocity of her conflict with colleagues regarding withdrawal of futile care) succinctly described this covenant when she said, 'I looked him in the eye and said, "I will take care of you", and that was it.' That was exactly how she saw it.

In its purest form, the covenantal ethic reduces the choice to life or death. Quality of outcome, or the burden of treatment vs. benefit, are not significant considerations.

While there is felt to be even the remotest chance of survival, the covenant makes it wrong to 'deprive' the person of this chance. It is inappropriate to consider what the patient might want (or would not accept) before the doctor has come to the conclusion that there is no chance of survival, 'no hope at all'.

It's not hard to see why surgeons might take this position. The 'best' doctors have the lowest mortality (who wants the surgeon who has the most post-operative deaths?).

The implication (or intensity) of the covenant can be influenced by the conversation that creates it. A very thoughtful, compassionate surgical colleague (who is incidentally an excellent surgeon) explained to me how important he found the last thing said to him by the patient (or family) before he operated.

When, during the consultation he had been implored to 'do his best', or was told that he was trusted to save the patient, he found it impossible to stop 'with a clear conscience', however badly things turned out. He felt he had been locked into a 'whatever it takes' path.

On the other hand, when the patient's or family's comments conveyed a theme of 'if we win that's good, but if not don't worry — we appreciate you trying', then he felt quite differently. He felt he had permission to stop if things went badly. He reflected that his patients probably had little understanding of the profound impact of their parting words when things did not go as well as hoped.

Death is the main factor we use to judge the quality of medicine. Journals report reductions in mortality as the main outcome-measure for medical research. Unless mortality is reduced, a new treatment is generally considered to have failed. Preventing death is the scientific measure of medical success.

This focus of medical care is so entrenched that it can be difficult to recognise how much it dominates all other considerations — until we come face-to-face with it for ourselves.

I often debrief friends and colleagues after their elderly parents have died. Many work in health care, and might be expected to understand the system. But they regularly tell me how difficult they found it was to get doctors to stop trying to cure, when a 'cure' was absolutely not their relative's wish or goal. They all reflect on how very difficult it must be for those who have neither their experience nor their confidence.

Vincent's story

I worked with Vincent many years ago when I was a young specialist. He was an older physician with a determined personality, who was used to getting his way.

Vincent would regularly, and proudly, state, 'I believe in never giving up', and he was certainly true to this. We often interacted because Vincent had many very sick, dying, deteriorating elderly patients under his care, whom he felt must all be admitted to the ICU (to get every possible medical intervention to prevent their dying).

We had many discussions because the ICU team frequently felt that unending escalation was not the best thing for these poor patients. But Vincent had no doubt. He didn't ask patients what they wanted, because he knew that they would want to do everything to live.

Vincent informed families with such an air of confidence that they invariably agreed. He had an affable, forceful personality, and his patients trusted him. Admission to ICU and massive treatment escalation was generally a 'done deal' before the ICU team knew anything about it. Any discussion to try to review the decision invariably resulted in confusion for the family and anger from Vincent.

There were occasional stark exceptions: I remember one particular elderly lady called Daisy. I went to see her after Vincent asked us to admit her to the ICU. Daisy was perfectly lucid, but very sick. When we asked her what she understood about what was happening, she told us that there had been 'talk going on about putting me on machines' — but that nobody had asked her. She told us that it wasn't going to happen. She said she had had a good life and didn't want to end it stuck on any machine. Daisy had no doubt about her wishes, was perfectly able to make her own decision, and could certainly communicate forcefully. She didn't come to ICU. She was a standout exception among so many others who were too ill, too confused, or too uncertain to influence events.

Once he got his patient into the ICU, Vincent would demand every treatment. For him, there were no limits. He was implacable. His deep religious conviction provided him with a profound duty to do everything to save life.

If he believed that there was the least chance that treatment could possibly work (even where the chance was vanishingly remote and the treatment was unpleasant), he would want it carried out. Misery, distress, and suffering resulting from ineffective treatment never seemed to be considerations for him. He didn't believe that patients had any right to decline, so he never offered any choice.

Vincent never seemed to regret poor outcomes in those we were able to pull through — observing that, in his experience, 'people have a great capacity to adapt'. He overruled any request from patients to forgo treatment on the grounds that 'people change their minds all the time'.

Inevitably, his patients had predictably awful deaths. Vincent seemed to have a knack for selecting people who had little to gain, and pushing them into treatment that had little to offer (and a lot to take). It was dreadful.

Vincent never tired of criticising the ICU team. He considered us to be 'miserable, nihilistic pessimists', and suggested that we didn't care about patients.

Then one evening, I had a call. Vincent had been brought into the emergency department, deeply unconscious. He had collapsed while walking his dog. Bystander CPR had been performed, and he had been defibrillated when the ambulance arrived. His heart had been restarted.

In view of the prompt resuscitation, we felt confident that Vincent would make a good recovery. But as the hours and days passed, the signs got worse and worse. A scan performed a week after the cardiac arrest showed massive, widespread damage. Everyone was shocked.

Three neurologists reviewed the scans and independently examined Vincent. All expressed grave concern. They agreed the damage was so severe that Vincent was not likely to survive. They agreed that if he were to survive then he would certainly be severely incapacitated, requiring long-term nursing-home care. All rated his chance of a 'good' recovery as nil.

We met with the family. All of them accepted the medical assessment — news that was clearly totally devastating. They were unanimous: 'Vincent would never, ever want to be kept alive if he couldn't recover to do things independently.' They said he would be furious if they went against his wishes. They had no doubt.

I sat quietly, reflecting on the direction of this

conversation. Was it possible that Vincent, who had advocated so fiercely, for so long, for so many, for so much inappropriate life-prolonging treatment … might not want the same for himself? Should we treat Vincent as he had treated so many others? Should we give him the choice that he had denied so many?

Vincent's wishes (as conveyed by his family) were accepted and respected.

He died quite quickly and peacefully, of a pneumonia that was left untreated.

Vincent's dual standards would not be totally unexpected. We think differently about ourselves than when we choose for others. Research shows that doctors regularly advocate for more treatment for their patients at the end of life than they would wish for themselves.

Things get more difficult when the illness and treatment are not seen as life threatening. Doctors find it particularly difficult when patients refuse (or their substitute declines on their behalf) a 'simple' treatment that the doctor believes is likely to work.

An example of such a 'simple' treatment would be the pinning of a fractured hip. This scenario has featured in several panel discussions that I have been involved in.

Hip fractures can often spark a train of events that ends in death for frail, elderly patients (with about half dying within one year of the fall). Many of us know someone for whom a hip fracture was the 'beginning of the end'. But fractures are not inevitably lethal, and death doesn't happen quickly. It would be unusual for us to consider someone with a fractured hip to be in the terminal phase of a terminal illness.

There is very good evidence that early surgical treatment of fractured hips (pinning them) saves lives. It is considered good practice to pin fractures quickly — and poor practice to delay surgery or not to surgically fix the fracture.

Where hips *don't* get pinned, there are two alternatives:

The first is 'conservative' treatment. This involves prolonged traction (many weeks in bed) while the fracture heals by itself.

The second is to palliate. This involves giving enough pain relief to ensure comfort while accepting death as an outcome. In this situation, early death is likely because these fractures are generally very painful, so the amount of pain relief required often results in such sedation and immobility that the patient ends up dying of pneumonia (but without distress or discomfort).

Conservative treatment for a hip fracture is generally a very poor option. Without being surgically fixed, these fractures are unstable and any movement causes severe pain (as the broken bone-ends rub on each other). This is a real problem. Anyone confined to bed needs to be turned regularly to prevent pressure sores — but turning causes terrible pain. The goal of conservative treatment is still cure. Since the goal is survival, everything needs to be done to minimise the chance of death — so regular turning is considered to be essential. Pain relief has to be limited in order not impair consciousness, movement, or coughing. *The goal of survival dominates all treatment decisions —* comfort is a secondary consideration.

The situation with palliation is quite different. In this case, the goal is comfort, and the priority is to ensure that there is no discomfort. There is no ambiguity. Whatever pain relief is required to achieve this goal is provided. The possibility that pain-relieving medication may cause or accelerate death is not accepted as reason to avoid giving it or to give less than required.

Defining the goal (or priority) is very important, but in many cases (not only in cases of hip fracture), the goals of treatment remain unclear and confused.

Audrey's story

June phoned me in tears. She is a tough lady who lived on a farm close to us.

June had brought her mum, Audrey, from interstate to a nursing home nearby so she could visit her regularly.

Audrey was mentally sharp, but she was very incapacitated, She was essentially bed bound. She talked wistfully about dying, but engaged with activities in the new nursing home and made friends.

Within a few months of arriving, Audrey fell and broke her hip. There was marked displacement. When the orthopaedic registrar came to get consent for surgery,

Audrey wasn't interested. She felt it would be a waste of time, money, and effort. She told him so. She asked for pain relief and to be allowed to die.

The registrar became angry. He asked why she had come to hospital if she didn't want treatment. Audrey pointed out it wasn't her choice and continued to make it clear that she did want treatment — she wanted proper pain relief. The registrar told her that, without an operation, she would be in agonising pain for weeks … but that it was her choice — and he walked off.

Audrey didn't get the pain relief she wanted because, she was told, it might kill her. It seemed to Audrey that she was going to be returned to the nursing home in severe pain.

It was then that June called me. She was understandably upset. I reassured her and called a colleague who is an excellent palliative-care specialist. He agreed to see Audrey and went over straight away.

Again, he advised Audrey that pinning her hip would be the most effective way to control pain, but she wasn't moved. He accepted her choice and respected her reasons. He identified her priority to avoid pain and clarified that prolonging life was not a priority for her. Audrey assured him that she was quite prepared for death.

Pain relief was administered until Audrey was comfortable. She was greatly relieved and, from that time, she never appeared to be in any pain.

Weeks of traction treatment would have had consequences that were exactly the opposite of what Audrey would have wanted. Surgery didn't fit with her priorities.

On another occasion, a different doctor recounted to me a similar case. This involved a severely demented patient who had also suffered a fracture. The family had refused consent for a pin and had requested palliation — just like Audrey. This doctor told how his patient had screamed every time she was turned for the next six weeks, until she died. He explained that he had been unwilling to give the requested pain relief because this would have caused her to develop 'complications'. He suggested that this proved that the family should have consented for the fracture to be pinned.

It seems that a patient-centric approach — to agree to a treatment plan based on a patient's priorities and goals — can be difficult.

Failure to identify a priority of care often results in the pursuit of an improbable cure dominating treatment decision-making. I will give you an example.

Mary's story

Mary was a retired primary-school teacher. She was a petite, neat lady who always did her best to present herself nicely.

When I first saw her, she had advanced colorectal cancer that had spread to her liver and lungs. She had been given a prognosis of three months some four months earlier (so she had done better than predicted) and was receiving palliative chemotherapy. Scans showed that her cancers were continuing to grow, despite treatment.

Mary had tripped and fallen as she got out of the car on her return home from a hospital visit for chemotherapy. She had broken several ribs. She hadn't wanted to go back to hospital and had taken herself to bed. Over the next 36 hours she had developed pneumonia on the side of her injury (because she was too sore to cough, and her immune defences were down due to her chemotherapy).

By the time Mary arrived back at hospital, her oxygen levels were very low, her breathing was shallow, and she was semi-conscious.

Mary's oncologist and her husband, Ken, were very keen that Mary should receive maximal treatment (including life support in ICU) to try to get her over this 'setback'.

As soon as we set eyes on her, it was clear to us that the cancer was taking a toll. Mary was dreadfully thin and she had virtually no muscle left. The pneumonia was serious and was progressing rapidly.

We needed to get Mary to take deep breaths and to cough if she were to survive. But she couldn't do either because of pain — she was in pain just with normal breathing.

We did what we could to relieve the pain without suppressing her ability to cough.

Local anaesthetic infused around the nerves in

her back helped, but not perfectly. Because the oxygen level in her blood was low, she needed an oxygen mask strapped to her face to deliver oxygen at increased pressure. She didn't like this.

Unfortunately, by this time the pain, the drugs, and the chest infection were causing Mary to be too confused to make any decisions for herself. She had to have her hands tied to stop her removing the mask and her drips.

Ken could see that Mary was distressed. He wanted her to be given medication to make her comfortable. He recognised that Mary had little time left and felt that being comfortable was 'the most important thing'. He was concerned that what was happening to her was 'torture'. He was sure she wouldn't want this, and hated seeing it.

We explained that our priority (as presented to us by Mary, Ken, and the oncology team when she was admitted to the ICU) was to do everything necessary to get Mary better (to try to 'cure' her).

We explained we could change direction to make comfort the number-one priority — and that this would be quite different to prioritising 'cure'.

Ken hadn't realised the extent that priorities might conflict, but understood how the aim to 'cure' the pneumonia had so quickly resulted in exactly what Mary didn't want (and what Ken didn't want for her, either).

Following a discussion with Mary's oncologist, the priority was changed to focus on comfort. We gave Mary enough medication to make her pain-free (given in repeated small doses until she appeared completely comfortable). The pneumonia worsened, and she died without further discomfort. Ken was with her.

Medical treatment designed to cure (particularly when intensive treatment is required) generally involves discomfort, often a lot of discomfort. Attempting to cure often limits the extent to which distressing symptoms can be relieved.

The view that we can pursue both cure and comfort at the same time (an 'each-way bet') often turns out to be a delusion.

Families play a big role in driving unpleasant, ineffective treatment (often more so than anyone may realise). The duty to save is such a strong motivation for families. 'Not trying' feels like abandonment, a failure; it feels so wrong. 'Not trying' makes everyone feel uncomfortable and readily attracts condemnation from onlookers and outsiders. The pressure to do something is profound.

A crisis makes things even more difficult for families. In a crisis, families regularly choose treatments that they consider to be inappropriate, including treatments that they know to be contrary to their relative's wishes. We see this often in our clinical practice and have confirmed it with our research —we have shown that we can get 100 per cent of substitutes to choose a treatment in a hypothetical crisis that they are certain that their relative would not want![2]

---

2   'Choosing Life Support for Suddenly Severely Ill Elderly Relatives.' C. F. CORKE, J. F. LAVERY, A. M. GIBSON. *Critical Care and Resuscitation* 2005; 7: 81-86

The power of the need to 'save' can easily overwhelm the wishes of competent patients. It is quite common to see frail, elderly patients who are quite adamant that they would *not* want a high-risk, low-benefit treatment change their mind after their family arrive. They generally explain their change of mind by saying that they will have treatment 'because my family want me to' or that they are 'doing it for the family'. This often seems coercive, unfair, and unwise.

CHAPTER 3

What about my wishes?

Wishes matter, but it can be difficult to get them heard.

Wanting to be saved is easy. 'To do whatever is required to save' is what everyone wants to do for you, needs to do, and is expected to do. It's what our medical system is designed to do. It's the default; it's what you get.

When we want to set limits, it's more difficult. The system is so intent and so comfortable to 'do' that it requires great confidence to convince everyone that it is OK not to.

Because doctors are so influential, and serious disease and death are so scary, wishes have to be very clear and very convincing to have any chance of having an effect. The key is to convey confidence.

Let's start out by illustrating just how hard it is to get others to follow a wish to stand back.

We recently conducted a study where we asked ordinary people to imagine they were in a room with an elderly person (we gave them no other information about this person). We told them that there was nobody else in the room and they couldn't call for help; however, we told them, there was a fully functioning automatic defibrillator on the wall.

Then we told them that the elderly person had collapsed with a cardiac arrest. They had to decide whether or not they would perform resuscitation.

The only things the participants had to guide them were different versions of statements from the elderly person's advance care plan (a formal document that records preferences for future treatment). We took the opinion that the elderly person wasn't keen to be resuscitated, and we wanted to find out what sort of statements most effectively reassured people not to resuscitate.

The first statement was simple and straightforward: 'Not for CPR.' This resulted in 85 per cent of the respondents not performing CPR. The statement is unambiguous and comes in the form of an instruction. Those who chose to resuscitate expressed concern that they didn't know enough about the person or their wishes to be confident.

The next statement included defining an acceptable outcome. We included a simple one: 'I would not want to be resuscitated if my heart stops, unless I can make a reasonable recovery. For me, a reasonable recovery means being able to communicate with my family.'

A lot of people make this sort of statement. It seems rational — rejecting a very poor outcome but still leaving opportunity for treatment. Unfortunately, it is rarely possible to confidently predict outcome, so it was not surprising to find that 75 per cent chose to resuscitate (in real life, where the pressure to act is greater, this would probably be nearer 100 per cent). Clearly, this statement is ineffective if the goal is to avoid resuscitation.

The next statement set stiff conditions: 'a full recovery'.

'I do not want to risk a poor end (as many of my friends have suffered). I would not want *any* attempt at resuscitation unless I can make a full recovery.'

Again, this sort of statement is common; it permits only really effective treatment with assured great outcomes. Here, 58 per cent chose *not* to resuscitate, mostly on the basis of being unable to guarantee a good outcome.

Next, we changed tack a bit, and tested some more 'emotional' pragmatic appeals.

'I have had a good life and am wearing out. I accept that I am going to die and want to get it over with. I do not want anyone to try to bring me back once I go.'

This provided significant reassurance, with 90 per cent electing not to resuscitate.

Finally, we added an appeal for wishes to be respected, including an appeal to love, to see how near to 100 per cent we could get.

'I accept that I am going to die and want to get it over with. I do not want anyone to try to bring me back once I go. I realise that it will be difficult to "do nothing", and I ask you to be strong. This is my choice and my responsibility. Please respect my right to make this decision as a mark of your respect and love (for those who do love me!). I have made my choice after much thought. I would not want anyone (family or doctor) to override my wish.'

Ninety-five per cent chose not to resuscitate, so we didn't quite get to 100 per cent. It seems that the remaining 5 per cent feel a binding duty to try because they can't be sure about the outcome or that the elderly person hadn't had a change of mind. It's difficult to know how it might be possible to reassure this 5 per cent in a way that would provide them with the confidence not to resuscitate.

So let's consider how to go about getting wishes about limits to be respected. Many people believe that, having thought about the issues and written down wishes, they can be confident that these wishes will be followed. It's not so simple.

Treating doctors, or concerned family, commonly ignore wishes in a crisis (often because they're unaware of their existence). Where wishes do get considered, they often get ignored in the pressure of the situation (and, as we will see later, many doctors think people actually want them to overrule expressed wishes in a crisis).

The system makes it difficult, too.

We rush people to hospital and implement treatment within minutes. Quality guidelines promote rapid, efficient treatment. There is no place for delay or deliberation. Now, stopping to think is liable to be regarded as an unnecessary, dangerous hesitation. Even negligent!

Brian's case illustrated several of the traps of planning as well as the influence of an 'efficient' medical system.

Brian's story

Brian was a 93-year-old farmer. His wife had died five years earlier. They had been married for 53 years, and he had loved her very much; she had been his best friend. He missed her dreadfully.

Brian continued living by himself in the same house on the farm where they had lived for over 50 years. Though frail, Brian remained active; he still drove a 1954 grey Ferguson tractor that he had meticulously restored.

Brian's daughter, Megan, lived nearby. She was busy with her law practice, but she regularly helped Brian with his shopping and other chores.

Brian had a few minor medical issues, but overall he was remarkably good for his age. He said that he valued his health 'such as it is', but he was concerned about what his future held. He completed an advance care plan and appointed his eldest son, Jack — 'because he's the eldest' — as his chosen substitute decision-maker.

In his written wishes, Brian stated that he didn't want CPR, didn't want any major treatment, and didn't want to go into a nursing home. He did want to be able to feed himself and to use the toilet by himself. In the final line, he said that he would accept treatment if he would still be able to interact with his family.

Brian didn't discuss his wishes with Jack because he felt that Jack was a 'busy man' and, anyway, Brian felt that Jack would 'know what to do'.

A couple of months after completing his plan, Brian

suffered a devastating stroke.

When he arrived at hospital, Brian was deeply unconscious.

Immediately, urgent scans (consistent with best-practice guidelines for stroke management) were performed. These included complex brain and vascular studies. They confirmed a large stroke, caused by clotting in a major artery supplying the left side of Brian's brain. The scans revealed that a significant area deep in the brain was already infarcted (dead) and a larger area was 'dying' but not yet dead. The report suggested that some of this 'dying' brain might be saved if Brian was to be given immediate clot-busting treatment.

The medical team assessed that it was likely that Brian would require nursing-home level of care, if he were to survive.

A choice needed to be made.

It was thought possible that Brian's life could be saved if the dying brain had its blood flow restored. The amount of brain that was already dead would leave him very incapacitated, but he could survive. If nothing was done, then half of Brian's brain would die, and it was very unlikely that he would survive. In that case, Brian could be given medications to ensure he suffered no distress.

Brian was unconscious, so the decision-making responsibility passed to Jack.

Jack had always found it very difficult to make decisions. He worried about everything. It had been a lifelong problem. His sister, Megan, was a lawyer and had always been better at weighing up situations and making decisions — but Brian hadn't appointed her. Jack felt the whole family showed Megan undue respect, and he resented this.

Jack had a copy of Brian's written wishes; as mentioned above, these started out identifying situations that Brian wouldn't want. Then there was the statement, 'I would accept treatment providing I am able to interact with my family.' It was difficult to reconcile this with the earlier wishes that were quite tough and quite clear. It suggested a more favourable attitude towards treatment, setting a low outcome bar ('being able to interact in some way — possibly as simple as a squeeze of the hand'). It suggested that Brian might have 'wanted to stay' to be with his family.

This last line in the plan resonated with Jack.

He chose clot-busting treatment, and signed the necessary consents.

The clot busting worked perfectly to restore blood flow, but, as predicted, Brian was left with very profound disability. He remained very confused and continued to be unable to make his own decisions. The doctors felt that it was appropriate to wait for some weeks to assess for any improvement. Jack agreed.

Brian had ongoing problems, and Jack consented to treatment for each of these. A PEG feeding tube was put through Brian's abdominal wall into his stomach (because his swallowing was seriously impaired by the stroke) and he was given powerful antibiotics for recurrent pneumonia (the stroke had so impaired Brian's cough and gag reflexes that his saliva dribbled down into his lungs. He wasn't able to cough it up and it festered — any food or drink did the same).

Eventually, Brian was discharged to a nursing home with an indwelling urinary catheter (because of urinary incontinence) and a nappy pad (because he couldn't control his bowels). He required a hoist to move him from bed to chair.

Brian was unable to talk or to write, which made communication difficult, but he was able to move one hand. He gestured with this, and, as time went on, he was able to convey simple messages.

From the start, Brian seemed deeply distressed and upset. A psychiatrist prescribed anti-depressants, but they didn't appear to help.

Brian regularly made gestures that suggested he wanted to die.

He eventually died of pneumonia after four months in the nursing home.

It's a sad story of a man who thought he had a plan.

Since Brian's death, we have met with Jack (at his request) to work through what happened.

This story illustrates lots of traps. Wishes have to be very clear. It is important to both identify situations that would be unacceptable (i.e., where death is preferable) and to explain how these wishes might be balanced against a small chance of success. Without such guidance for decision-makers, wishes to avoid a bad outcome are likely to be ignored in favour of a gamble for an unlikely cure — with wishes about what is not wanted being viewed as vague 'hopes' and 'desires', rather than as an important instruction.

Brian contributed some ambiguity. His plan said that he didn't want to become dependent in a nursing home, but he hadn't said that he would rather *die* than to go into a home. Few of us 'want' to go into a nursing home, but sometimes there is simply no choice. The same applies to his wishes about feeding and using the toilet — would he rather die? We can't know with certainty from what he wrote down.

Then there is the statement — 'I would accept treatment if I am able to interact with family.' A lot of people put a final 'softening' statement in their plan. It may reflect a lack of firm commitment to set limits, but more often, it appears it is added to placate others (the family, the doctor, or the person assisting with the writing of the plan). It seems that people can also find it difficult to accept great determination in plans that others make, and feel the need to encourage the person writing the plan to 'water it down' a bit.

The inclusion of this sort of statement (identifying a 'low bar' that *is* wanted) can easily invalidate everything in the plan about what is *not* wanted. Jack certainly acknowledged that Brian's statement about being able to interact with family had had this effect on him.

Jack also explained how he felt pushed into agreeing to the treatment because he felt that the doctors were really keen to give the clot-busting drug. He felt he had been asked to consent to something that had already been decided. He thought that had he refused consent, it would have meant that he was 'being difficult'. Jack liked to please — it wasn't in his nature to be difficult.

Looking back, Jack bitterly regretted having agreed to treatment. He felt responsible for everything that ensued. Megan was furious with him, suggesting he had 'totally failed' in his responsibility. The relationship between the siblings broke down.

Jack wished the doctors had not offered the treatment when his dad first arrived in hospital. He wished the doctors had 'at least' looked at Brian's advance care plan then (apparently, there was a copy in Brian's medical record, but it was never raised with Jack).

Jack appeared crushed, clearly damaged by the experience. We organised counselling for him, and he hasn't come back to see us, so I hope he is now OK and has been able to come to terms with what happened.

Thinking about circumstances where we believe that life would *not* be worth living can be difficult. It involves thinking about living in a way we would consider utterly unacceptable, by necessity an unpleasant task, as it involves thinking about suffering and dying. It's human nature to try to avoid thinking about bad or difficult things.

Often, thinking about what is important to us to 'make

life worth living' seems easier (because it involves thinking about good things). Understanding what makes life worth living for an individual provides insight into what sort of person they are, and how they think about their life. But we shouldn't presume that losing the ability to do these things would necessarily make life '*not* worth living', so the discussion needs to continue to establish whether the loss of things that make life worth living means that this person would prefer to be dead if these important things were lost. Unfortunately, many discussions stop at a description of what we find nice about life, which is interesting, but doesn't help decision-making!

Identifying unacceptable outcomes goes straight to the point, and some people prefer to be straightforward. There are wide ranges of outcomes (and treatment experiences) that many people suggest as being unacceptable to them.

'Not being a vegetable' is probably the most common thing that people say they won't accept, and is possibly the least useful statement. Obviously, it describes a poor level of function, but for a doctor, being a 'vegetable' would (presumably) mean to be in a Persistent Vegetative State (PVS) — a diagnosis that requires months of observation before it can be made. Looked at this way, this wish provides doctors with little help for decision-making at the time of crisis. It is also difficult to know exactly how little function the person making the plan would consider a 'vegetable' might have (if they don't mean to describe the specific medical condition).

Another common limit is 'being unable to communicate with my family'. We have thought about this one a bit already. Communication is a broad concept. For some, being able to communicate would involve the ability to engage in high-level debate and discussion — but for others, it might include a squeeze of the hand, a blink of an eye, or a tiniest suggestion of a smile. These simple things are often seen to convey great meaning and to represent a very profound sort of communication.

Unless it is otherwise stated, 'communication' is generally interpreted as meaning these more basic, simple (emotional) sort of interactions.

Recent research from Cambridge (in 2008)[3] has pushed the bounds of what it means to be able to 'communicate' even further. This group examined patients with a diagnosis of PVS, using functional-brain scanning, and demonstrated that in some patients, particular areas of the brain 'lit up' in response to questions. This created lots of interest, because the researchers were demonstrating communication with patients who were otherwise totally unresponsive. This greatly extends the limits of what it may mean to be 'able to communicate', quite possibly beyond what most people might intend when writing this in a plan.

Looking at a few examples of actual phrases from actual plans can help us to consider how easily they might be interpreted (or misinterpreted) at the time of a future crisis

---

3   Owen et al. 'Residual auditory function in persistent vegetative state: a combined PET and
    fMRI study.' *Neuropsychol Rehabil.* 2005 Jul-Sep;15(3-4):290-306.

(when the person writing them would be unable to explain exactly what they meant).

Putting lots of things together is common but confusing:

I would not want treatment if I cannot feed myself and I can't go to the toilet on my own and I can't recognise my family.

Would *all* these conditions need to be present in order for this plan to be enacted?

When I am close to death, I would not want any treatment that would simply prolong my dying.

This sort of plan sets a minimal bar. The first statement identifies that this only applies in the period just before death (and only once the dying process has been recognised and accepted). And the second sets a minimal limit that doctors and family are likely to adopt anyway (without needing any guidance from the patient). Stating this wish does nothing to assist with difficult treatment choices earlier in the course of deterioration.

I would not want to be resuscitated.

This goes some way to being useful, but it conveys inadequate explanation. What precisely does it mean? Does it exclude a witnessed arrest when there is a defibrillator available and the expected outcome is full recovery? Does it convey fear of a poor outcome, along with a desire not to risk this by accepting resuscitation? Or does it convey a readiness to die and a desire not to be 'brought back'? The statement itself doesn't tell us.

I would not want to end up in a nursing home.

Again, this goes some way to being useful, but again it conveys inadequate explanation. Few of us would *want* to be in a nursing home, but does this statement imply a *preference to die* rather than to be in a nursing home? It is important to know.

Furthermore, it can be difficult to predict outcomes with certainty. How should this plan be interpreted where a patient is highly likely to end up needing nursing-home placement, but where this is not certain?

This is a useful starting statement, but it needs more clarification.

No heroics or *No unnecessary medical treatment.*

Both of these statements convey a suggestion that the patient has some limits — but both are wide open to interpretation. Again, these are useful starting statements but require more explanation and clarification.

I don't want to be a burden on my family.

The desire not to become a burden on our children as we become increasingly dependent is very common. It is clearly something that many people see as important. The wish not to burden our children reflects a popular narrative that our role as parents is to set up the next generation, to do our best for them, and this does not involve dragging them down as we age.

This directly conflicts with the duty that families feel to look after relatives: to 'accept the burden of caring' and to do so without complaint. From the family's perspective, their relative can only be a burden if they consider them to be a burden. Where the family see value in the person, and recognise their duty to care, then this person can never be considered to be a burden — in this view, caring is a duty and a privilege.

The judgmental nature of this assessment makes it very difficult for families to contemplate, and certainly to openly discuss, the concept of burden.

Paradoxically, the guilt and discomfort associated with accepting that someone you love *is* a burden may encourage families to strongly advocate for life prolongation — just to make it clear to everyone that they *do* care.

But it is not all bad. Clear statements can be very powerful. On their own (i.e., not all linked together), statements about being able to toilet independently, being unable to feed oneself, and to accept (or not accept) nursing-home placement can be useful. These outcomes can often be predicted with reasonable confidence quite early, and knowing that these are unacceptable outcomes can certainly help decision-making.

Statements that express how someone generally thinks about life and death can help, too — how someone feels about suffering, longevity, quality of life, and dignity. How they see hope and struggle. Whether they feel human life is sacred, or indeed, whether they think dying is their choice to make. These things convey a view of the world that can help predict choices at the end of life.

Having thought about things in general terms, it is probably time to focus on how to create a 'good plan'.

There is often little overlap between the ambiguous wishes that most people feel comfortable to write down and the unambiguous instruction that those needing to make these difficult decisions look for. In my experience, plans that convey humanity and 'talk to the heart' seem to work best (from both perspectives).

I won't claim that my plan is perfect, or that it would be appropriate for you to copy it — but I share it here to provide an example of what I think a good, clear plan might look like:

I am very happy to receive any treatment that is likely to restore me to good health.

I would rather die than to be cared for in a nursing home. I absolutely do not want you to have to care for me if I can't do everyday things for myself and I would utterly resent burdening any of you (and I think I would be utterly frustrated and would be awful to look after).

Please don't be tempted to keep me alive if it is likely that I can't do any of the things that you know matter so much to me, including being independent, walking, and working.

A plan like this leaves little room for ambiguity and should be easy to apply in lots of different clinical situations.

There is another approach that does not involve 'forms' (though it can provide a useful supplement to a formal plan). This is probably the most meaningful and powerful way to express wishes. It involves writing a letter to the family (ideally, separate versions to each member). Many people find this easier than completing formal documents.

A personal letter talks to the heart. It starts loved ones on a journey to acceptance; it affirms love and connection, and it evokes all those things that are so important.

Every letter will be different, every memory highly personal and special. But the intent to connect is the same. Here is an example of the way an effective message might look (a letter that one of my patients wrote):

Dearest Joy,

I am writing you a special letter to tell you some things that are important to me.

I want to tell you that I have had a fabulous life, and you have been a very important part of that. I realise that it is coming towards the end and I accept that.

I want to share some of my feelings and special memories with you. The first time I held you, just seconds after you were born, was the happiest day of my life. I always remember how bright and how perfect your eyes were. I loved you from that moment.

I was so proud the day you got your diploma, you worked so hard for that. All those evenings working on the old kitchen table, you doing your study and me doing mine. Remember the demarcation line where my papers couldn't pass!

And when we went to Hobart on the bicycles; that was special too.

There are so many good things that I remember.

It's all been so wonderful, but I am wearing out, and my illness is slowly winning. I know I can't go on forever and I'm concerned about how this end bit will be. I don't want it to be messy. You know I want to go without fuss and I hope I can. I have always liked Auntie Jean's saying: 'it's better to leave the party before everyone wishes you'd go and while they want you to stay'. That's what she did, and I hope I can, too.

When I am very ill, and it looks like I may die, I hope you will carefully listen to each other and the doctors, and that you will come to an agreement together based on my wishes and concerns (that I hope you all know well by now!). If agreement is not possible (and I realise these things can be difficult), then I want Graham (as my legally appointed medical decision-maker) to decide for me. I'd ask you to respect his decision.

I know your decisions may hasten my death, which is fine; no one should feel guilty. Please let me go. I think that letting go is the deepest sort of love.

I want adequate pain medication even if it may hasten death (particularly if it does!). I don't want anyone to suggest that I may have received too much pain medication *(but please do ask for me to be given more if you have any concern that I may be uncomfortable).*

I do not want my life extended if my outlook is grim. Please don't suggest that the treatment I get may not be enough! Easy treatment that is very likely to work is fine, but please don't push it.

I don't want to be any worse than I am now; if the doctors can't confidently predict a quick and full recovery then please keep me comfortable and let me go.

With all my love, Dad xxxxxx

A letter like this can easily say it all in a very powerful way. Evoking special memories is a particularly powerful way to connect. Humour, especially black humour, evokes our humanity and bonds us.

I think of letters like this as an advance care plan — but one presented in a different way than the more formal sort.

There are other unconventional ways to plan. Antonio's was one of these:

Antonio's story

Antonio was a much-loved husband and grandfather of eight.

He played a regular Wednesday game of golf with his longstanding friend, Paulo. They had done this weekly for 30 years.

Although both were well, they knew that they were getting on in years. It was a regular topic of conversation, as they worried about how their final days might be.

A mutual friend had suffered a severe stroke from which he had never recovered. This had left a strong impression on both of them.

Together, they made a pact that if either of them were to suffer a catastrophic event, but were to survive, the other would promise to take them 'off the machine' so they could die (ignoring the consequences!). They had told their families of their pact. It was extreme but resolute. Importantly, it carried a clear message of wishes and determination.

Almost exactly one year later, Antonio collapsed on the golf course, just as he was about to drive on the 14th hole. He had suffered a cardiac arrest.

Paulo quickly started resuscitation, with the help of other golfers who were nearby. Someone called an ambulance, but it took some time to get there as they were far out on the course. Once they arrived, the ambulance crew restarted Antonio's heart and took him to hospital.

Sadly, by the next day, it was obvious that Antonio had suffered severe brain damage. It was too soon to be certain about any improvement, but it was extremely likely that Antonio would be severely disabled and would never return to independence.

The family was told of the situation. They asked about the chance of a good recovery. The neurologist told them that, in his opinion, there was 'no realistic chance of a good recovery'. He explained that Antonio could recover to some extent, but he couldn't be sure of how much.

The family accepted the assessment of a bad outcome. They were quite certain that Antonio would only want to fully recover and would not want to recover poorly.

There seemed no doubt that Antonio was much loved and respected. There were a lot of tears.

Both families were well aware of the 'pact'; they even joked about it. There was discussion about the content of the Italian food parcels that they would need to send to Paulo in prison.

We assured Paulo that he need not worry about being jailed, because we would (and should) only treat Antonio if that was what he would have wanted us to do — and in the current situation, it didn't sound like he would have.

The family, with Paulo, agreed without hesitation that Antonio would not want us to strive to keep him alive, as it was virtually certain that he would not recover.

We took Antonio off the life support. He breathed ineffectively for a few minutes, and then he died.

Antonio had done none of the legal or formal advance care planning that is generally advocated. He hadn't appointed Paulo (or anyone else) to be his formal decision-maker. He hadn't written anything down.

Despite this, he had convincingly conveyed his wishes in his own (unusual) way that had made everyone completely confident that by stopping, they were doing exactly what he would have wanted.

How substitutes behave is vitally important. Many do a fantastic job. Some really stand out. Vlado was one of those:

Kreso's story

Kreso had emigrated from Croatia in the 1950s. He had a successful life and raised a loving family.

Though he loved his family, Kreso appointed his long-term best friend, Vlado, to be his medical decision-maker. Kreso explained that he chose Vlado because he was a successful businessman who was used to making difficult decisions. He felt Vlado would be able to make decisions without too much emotion (in contrast to his family). Kreso felt that after so many years they understood each other.

Late in life, Kreso developed a number of chronic conditions that frustrated him. Eventually, he suffered a major stroke and couldn't communicate.

The treating neurologist spoke to the family and to Vlado. He clearly explained the situation and mentioned the possibility of a treatment that he felt had some small chance of improving things, but which also carried some risks.

The family were concerned. Vlado asked if they

could have a second opinion. This was arranged. It confirmed what the family had already been told.

Vlado encouraged all the family to share their thoughts. He was careful not to exclude anyone or to suggest that as he was the appointed decision-maker, it didn't matter what anyone else felt.

Finally, after listening to everyone, Vlado explained that it was his responsibility to make a final decision, because that was what Kreso had asked him to do.

He explained that if he were in Kreso's position he felt that he would want to try the treatment, but because of his understanding of Kreso, he felt that his friend would not want to go through this for an unlikely benefit — and ongoing ill health.

The family deferred to Vlado. They expressed their support for his authority and interpretation. Vlado conveyed the decision to decline the treatment to the neurologist, who accepted the decision.

Kreso's condition continued to deteriorate. He died 24 hours later with his family by his side.

The family expressed relief that Vlado had taken the responsibility of having to make an 'impossible' decision from them.

Vlado said he was proud to have been able to help his great friend by accepting this task. He spoke quietly of the wonderful friend Kreso had been, and how much he would miss him. He spoke of his new responsibility to support Kreso's family.

Decision-making can be very difficult, especially when it involves someone who is dearly loved. It is important to consider this when choosing whom to appoint:

Kostas's story

Kostas came from Cyprus with his parents when he was five years old. He did well at school and went on to establish a successful business.

At 24, he had married Eleni. She was 10 years older, very sensible, fiercely loyal and practical. She brought stability to his life. It was a good match, and they were very happy together.

All was well until Kostas had a routine check-up just before his 59th birthday. The tests revealed that he was in severe kidney failure, and worse, the cause was a myeloma (a cancer of antibody-producing cells).

He started dialysis and treatment for his myeloma. Unfortunately, his myeloma proved highly resistant to treatment. There was no return of his kidney function.

Kostas suffered a variety of serious side effects from increasingly desperate treatment measures. Eventually, he got pneumonia, and ended up on a mechanical ventilator to support his breathing and a dialysis machine to support his kidneys. He needed regular blood transfusions.

Weeks passed without improvement; indeed, rather than getting better, Kostas got worse. He was a shadow of the man who had gone for a simple check-up. He was far too sick to be able to make any decisions for himself.

By this time, he was in no state to tolerate any treatment for his myeloma, which was progressing rapidly. As he got sicker, we realised that we were never going to be able to get him off the ventilator.

There was a general agreement between all the medical teams that ongoing life support was inappropriate — it would prolong an existence that was causing Kostas great distress, without offering any chance of survival.

Eleni was asked for her agreement to the plan to stop treatment. She responded categorically that she 'would never agree, could never agree' to let Kostas die.

She was adamant. It went on for days. Numerous attempts to persuade Eleni failed. Previously, she had been constant in her visits, but now these became infrequent.

I met with Eleni and listened carefully to try to understand her position. She reiterated that she could never agree to let Kostas die. I asked her to tell me more. She explained that she felt that she was being asked to be 'part of the panel that condemns him' and 'to be the one who pulls the trigger'. She felt everyone was making her take responsibility. She felt it was unfair.

I asked her whether she felt Kostas was going to get better (she didn't) and whether she thought he was suffering (she was certain that he was). She felt it was awful. It was the reason she couldn't bear to come in — 'to sit there just to watch him suffer'.

I asked how she'd feel if I were to make the decision.

She said that was exactly what she wanted. She said it was our responsibility as doctors. I asked if she would be able to accept it if we decided to stop.

She said she'd accepted it for a long time.

Many older people choose to delegate all decision-making at the end of life to their doctor — believing that 'my doctor will know what to do' — rather than stating their own wishes or passing the responsibility to their family. This reflects tremendous respect for the doctors' decision-making (which is often unfounded), but it also generally relates to one particular trusted doctor, who may well not be involved when the time comes to make a decision.

Delegating to doctors relies on a model of medicine that has now become rather uncommon. It evokes a doctor who intimately knows the person and their wishes. It presumes that this doctor will be the treating doctor in a crisis (and will be the only one making decisions). Modern medicine isn't like this. It is now common for many different doctors to be involved in the care of a single patient — and a family doctor is rarely involved in decisions that occur in crisis, in hospital.

When patients, their families, and doctors are tackling end-of-life choices, they are guided (sometimes unwittingly) by two main principles.

The first is autonomy. This is our right to exist as an independent entity and to be permitted to make our own decisions.

The second is beneficence. This is where someone acts in the 'best interest' of someone else. The person doesn't get to choose for themselves, but a decision is made for them that is felt to be the best choice.

In the past, most medical decisions were based on beneficence. More recently, a person's right to control their own life, to do as they wish (even where others disagree), is considered to be very important.

When someone is unconscious (or otherwise incapable of making their own decisions), there are two ways that autonomy can be preserved:

The first is to follow any 'explicit wishes' that the person may have communicated. These could be written instructions or something that they have clearly said.

The second method is 'substituted judgment'. Here, the decision is made based on how the person might think (that is, the answer they would be predicted to give under the circumstances).

Beneficence (acting in 'best interest') involves acting in a way that best benefits the patient (often regardless of what the patient may have said they would want). It assumes that patients may need to be 'protected' by others who will make better decisions for them.

It is not always obvious what course of action would actually be in a patient's best interests.

There are plenty of examples of actions — taken because they are thought to be in someone's best interest — that are deeply resented by that person. When our autonomy is removed, we often become deeply dissatisfied, even when the choices made for us may appear reasonable to others (anyone with teenage children will understand this!).

It can be difficult to see how something as awful as death can ever be in a person's best interests. But where existing quality of life is poor, the burden of treatment of disease is high, or when treatment offers little or no benefit, then the balance of harms and benefits can easily make a peaceful death a preferable choice.

Despite increasing respect for autonomy, it is important to recognise that we are never truly autonomous. We rarely make decisions in a vacuum, particularly in regard to important things (like dying). We all live in a complex web of relationships, where our decisions are very much dependent on these relationships. We are influenced by a desire not to disappoint — to conform.

Enabling people to decide for themselves requires that clear, balanced, honest, and accurate information is provided to them (enabling them to make an informed decision). Many doctors and families find it difficult to provide this information. However, sick patients often desire far greater frankness than everyone realises:

Sylvia's story

Sylvia was a 76-year-old who underwent surgery for stomach cancer. Sadly, at operation it was obvious that the cancer had spread so widely that it was inoperable.

Her type of cancer was known to be highly resistant to other treatments (chemotherapy and radiotherapy). It was very serious.

The surgeon decided that it would be best not to tell Sylvia about the extent of her cancer until she had fully recovered from the operation.

But Sylvia didn't recover; she developed a serious pneumonia. She went into respiratory failure. The surgical team asked Sylvia if she wanted to be put on a breathing machine should her breathing continue to deteriorate.

Unaware of the situation with her cancer (she presumed the operation had dealt with it), Sylvia said that she wanted the breathing machine.

For the next four weeks, until her death, Sylvia remained on life support. The antibiotics worked, but she never had the strength to get off the ventilator. She didn't heal and her operation wound broke down. The surgeon felt it was a sad end, but he repeatedly pointed out that it had been her choice to come to the ICU.

Treatment decisions need to be properly informed, and it is not appropriate that any information that is vital to the decision should be withheld.

Proper autonomous decision-making (when we make decisions for ourselves) requires that *all* reasonable choices are offered and discussed. All the information required to make the decision should be provided.

Ideally, options should to be presented carefully, ensuring that they address that individual's values and priorities.

Some people suggest that personal decision-making is so open to influence that it can't ever be relied upon. They may have a point, but the alternative — letting other people judge what is in our best interest — is generally even less reliable.

Paternalism is a type of 'best interest' approach, but is subject to influence by the views of the person making the decision (paternalism roughly translates as 'father knows what is best for you'). When we presume to know what is best for another person, it is very easy to get it wrong, because we don't fully understand the perspectives of the other person.

Despite the risks, there *are* some advantages when someone experienced (such as a doctor) makes a best-interest decision for us. There is no need for the person involved to hear all the facts and choices (which may be distressing and/or overwhelming) or to struggle with the decision.

Decisions made by doctors generally involve less emotion and may be more logical. Doctors often have extensive experience of what has happened in other, similar, cases on which to base their decision.

However, when doctors make a best-interest decision on behalf of a patient, they need a deep understanding of their patient's wishes and values. This can be achieved through a long association (for instance, a GP caring for a patient over many years) or a detailed conversation exploring aspects of the person's values, fears, and wishes.

A lifelong doctor–patient relationship has become unusual, and a doctor taking the time to discuss values or fears with patients is also pretty rare. Consequently, doctors often know little of how their patients feel, and this makes paternal decision-making unreliable.

On the other hand, patients often have inadequate (or inaccurate) information on which to base their decisions, and most commonly make decisions based on an overly optimistic assessment on what is ahead (particularly as things get bad, and a frank assessment becomes uncomfortable for doctors to convey).

Neither approach is really good. In practice, the best solution seems to be to share the decision between the doctor, patient, and family. This includes aspects of autonomy and best interest (we call this 'shared decision-making').

Reports suggest that more than 80 per cent of people appreciate some form of shared process when confronted by difficult medical treatment decisions. This involves negotiation. The doctor provides information about the medical situation and the prognosis, and may express an opinion on the best course of management (from a medical perspective). The patient (or the family) provides insight into the patient's values, wishes, fears, and experiences — how they think, who they are, and how the treatment or outcome is expected to affect them.

Following this sharing of information, discussion

proceeds towards an agreed treatment decision. Ideally, all this happens in an atmosphere of mutual trust and respect. The healthcare team shares the burden of decision-making, reducing the chance that the family will feel the whole weight of responsibility, which can be substantial in the case of a decision to let a loved one go.

The success of shared decision-making depends on the willingness of doctors to make time for these discussions, and for everyone to understand their role in the process.

Where the doctor makes 'best interest' decisions based on his (or her) own strong personal 'ethical' views, this can be incompatible with good, shared decision-making. It can easily result in decisions that are resented by patients and families. When a doctor has beliefs that are quite different to those of their patient, most authorities believe that the doctor has an obligation to be open about this and to provide access to an alternative doctor who has no such constraint.

Some legislation incorporates clauses requiring doctors to withdraw or withhold treatment *only* when they consider the request to be 'reasonable' (as a safeguard against unreasonable requests and to protect doctors). Some doctors apply a rather limited interpretation to the word 'reasonable', taking this to mean a choice with which they agree — everything else being considered to be 'unreasonable'. It is likely that the intent of these clauses was to protect from very *un*reasonable decisions — that is, decisions that clearly differ from the expressed wishes of the patient, or where demands are made with which (almost) nobody in the general or medical community could or would concur.

In practice, it is prudent for families to question why a doctor considers a request to be 'unreasonable' (or simply ignores a request), as the definition of unreasonableness can be so subjective.

As we consider decision-making, it is important to recognise that people have quite different opinions about how their treatment decisions should be made.

A study that asked seriously ill patients how they wanted doctors to be involved in their treatment decisions showed that there is no one 'right' approach:

Ten per cent want to leave the decision entirely to their doctor; 9 per cent want their doctor to decide, but take their opinion into account; 32 per cent think that they and their doctor should work together, on an equal basis, to arrive at a decision ('shared'); 24 per cent want to make the final decision for themselves, after considering their doctor's opinion, while just 16 per cent want to make the treatment decision alone (without any input from their doctor). The remaining 10 per cent were uncertain.

This range of opinion has also been observed among terminal cancer sufferers, where 52 per cent wanted to share decision-making with their doctors, and 15 per cent wanted their doctor to make the decision (including a decision to stop treatment) on their behalf.

Clearly, these are very different expectations. It seems that *how* the decision is to be made needs to be negotiated before the actual decision-making process starts.

It also seems that families have a similar range of expectations about how decisions will be made.

Up till now, we have thought about dying in terms of how we might respond to sudden serious deterioration at the end of life. This has been our focus because this is how most people die — dying *of* something. Most of us want to go on until something clearly bad happens, and then we want to stop. We have been considering where that point is, and how we can help everyone recognise when we get there.

However, it is appropriate here to review the role of active assisted dying or voluntary euthanasia. This means intentionally taking something in order to end our life. Clearly, this removes all worry about a potentially bad end that we can't control – voluntary euthanasia is all about control.

It's a very topical subject, and some advocates might suggest that much of what we have been discussing would be redundant, if euthanasia were legal and available.

Nancy's story

I didn't realise at the time, but I first witnessed euthanasia (or more accurately, voluntary active dying) when I was about 10 years old.

It involved Nancy, a lovely, eccentric lady who lived next door. Nancy was a spinster, who lived alone in a huge house with a beautiful garden. My brother and I regularly went for tea, when she would invariably have a new game for us to play together. I particularly remember playing pick-up-sticks with her in her kitchen one cold winter's afternoon, as well as croquet on the lawn in summer.

We were always excited to be invited and we always had a good time. These were happy memories.

Nancy was the first person I remember having cancer. Hers was an aggressive breast cancer that had already spread widely by the time she was diagnosed.

Nancy was frank with us in the way that some adults are, and that children seem to appreciate. I can't recall being in the least disturbed — we realised it wasn't good, but I can't honestly remember being upset. I do vividly recall Nancy telling us about the brain surgery she had had through her nose. You might feel this was a terrible thing for an adult to tell young children, but it was in Nancy's nature to be forthright, and we didn't mind. Actually, we thought it was wonderfully gruesome.

Like most boys of our age, we were fascinated with ancient Egypt, especially how they removed the brains from the dead during mummification by pushing a metal probe up the nose, cracking through the thin bone at the top of the nose, and getting into the brain — and then sucking the brain out through a hollow tube.

Now here was Nancy, living right next door, who had actually had it done to her! It was so cool.

From our perspective, Nancy's illness changed nothing except to raise her to mythical hero status.

Our visits continued. It got even better when Nancy arranged a really big children's party. It was a huge summer garden party with lots of children, many of whom we had never seen before. In my mind, I can still see the roundabout in the garden and all of us sitting on the grass, watching an amazingly skilled magician who enthralled us all. It was undoubtedly my very best childhood party ever.

A few days later, there was more excitement. Lots of police arrived at Nancy's house ('lots' in our small town wasn't very many, but there were several officers and they came in a police car with lights, so we were very impressed).

Now we were living next door to a crime scene.

We felt like detectives as we collected every bit of information we could to try to find out what was going on. We discovered that Nancy had died 'under suspicious circumstances'. We heard she had killed herself by taking all of her tablets, all at once. Apparently, her cancer had been advancing rapidly, despite her operation.

Some adults around us suggested that taking her own life showed that Nancy was weak and unwilling to fight, unable to 'take it'. But others disagreed, suggesting that it showed what a strong and determined woman Nancy really was. I don't recall us having any view at the time, one way or the other. We were too young to think deeply and, to be honest, we were totally overwhelmed by the thrill of it all.

(NOTE: Pituitary ablation was a common treatment at the time, in the early 1960s. Removal of the pituitary gland reduced oestrogen secretion, and this helped control some hormone-dependent breast cancers. With the development of highly specific oestrogen-blocking drugs, the operation is no longer done for this purpose.)

Reflecting on it now, I think I can understand how much of a threat Nancy's advancing cancer must have presented to her dignity and independence — things I suspect would have been vitally important to her. I can understand how it might have seemed perfectly logical to Nancy to 'get out' before she lost too much of what mattered most in her life. I doubt that even the most fantastic palliative care would have been able to satisfy her needs and allay her fears.

Many might conclude that the current situation (going on and on from one failing treatment to the next) is so unacceptable that voluntary euthanasia (voluntary assisted dying) represents a better solution — possibly the only reliable solution.

Unfortunately, this may be rather optimistic.

Voluntary euthanasia relies on the unswerving determination of the person who is requesting that their life be terminated. Clearly, this needs steely determination. But this is exactly the sort of clarity that we require to set limits as we confront serious, life-limiting illness, and it is this that we so rarely see.

We already have the right, and the legal support, to refuse life-saving treatment — we just shy away from doing it. Society wants euthanasia to help us face our concerns about our eventual dying.

Euthanasia has been legalised in the Netherlands, Switzerland, Oregon (USA), in Quebec (Canada), and, more recently, in Canada as a whole. In each case, few people use it. Of those who do 'sign up', as many die (of their disease) without taking the lethal drug as complete the process and take the drug.

Overall, legal euthanasia accounts for less than 1 per cent of all deaths in those places where it has been permitted. While it may be very important to the 1 per cent, and its possibility may be reassuring to a larger number, it still leaves 99 per cent to go on to die of some disease or other. How far we push on (or want to push on) remains the vital question for those of us who end up this way (and the ongoing topic of this book).

Rather than focusing too much on euthanasia, it might be more useful if we were to think more about 'dysthanasia'. The word 'dysthanasia' comes from the Latin '*dys—*' meaning unpleasant or distressing and '*—thanasia*' meaning death. Dysthanasia does not appear in *The Oxford Concise Dictionary*, something that might help explain why it has been such a difficult concept for us to recognise.

Dysthanasia might specifically identify situations where medical treatment actively and unnecessarily contributes to the unpleasantness of dying. It is something that we could probably all agree that we are against. Being sensitive to the possibility should help us to avoid it.

The next cases illustrate how decision-making about treatment at the end of life contributes to a 'good' or a 'bad' death.

Rita's story

Rita was from a small rural town where she ran a milk bar with her husband. She was a tough, chubby, cheerful hard worker.

Tragically, in late middle age, Rita developed a rapidly progressive dementia. The family managed to keep her at home until her kidneys unexpectedly failed.

Her kidney failure quickly progressed to the level where dialysis was required.

Because of the dementia, Rita was unable to understand the concepts required to make decisions, and the situation was discussed with her family.

They were divided.

Some felt that Rita would 'never want any of this', while others reported how determined Rita had been throughout her life and how she could 'put up with anything' — they felt she would want treatment.

Some mentioned things that Rita seemed to enjoy, such as food and flowers, to justify keeping her alive with dialysis. She certainly seemed happy most of the time and to appreciate little things.

Others cited her loss of interaction, loss of dignity, and poor quality of life as justification for not 'subjecting' her to dialysis ('subjecting' was the word they used).

One younger son made it particularly clear that he could 'never let Mum go'. He suggested that she should 'be given a chance'. He seemed very forceful, and the rest of the family deferred to him.

Medical staff felt uncomfortable to withhold dialysis in the face of family disagreement. Rita was started on the dialysis program.

Family tensions increased as they disputed who cared most (those who wanted dialysis or those who didn't). Each group accused the other of being 'heartless'.

Nursing staff expressed incredulity. They felt that Rita was uncooperative with dialysis and seemed distressed by the process.

Things continued in this way for some time, until Rita suffered a cardiac arrest during dialysis. CPR was performed, but it proved ineffective and Rita died.

Medical staff felt that treatment had pushed on for far too long, and they blamed this on the family.

The family blamed doctors because they felt dialysis should never have been offered.

Rita could have helped if she had said what she didn't want, or how far she would want to go, before dementia overtook her.

Bill's story

Bill had had a long and successful life. He had worked as an accountant and had a long career in local council as a financial controller. At one stage, he had been elected mayor.

Bill had been married to Agnes for 60 years. They had a daughter, Teresa, who was a nurse.

In his early 80s, Bill began to display signs of dementia. Appropriate investigation failed to identify any reversible cause. Despite medication to slow progression, he steadily deteriorated.

Bill was still able to look after himself to some extent, but his memory was poor. In his lucid moments, Bill repeatedly expressed concern about his memory and regularly expressed the hope that 'something would get him' before he 'really lost it'.

One morning, Bill woke with severe pain across his chest. He wasn't very clear when he described the pain, but Agnes and Teresa worked out that the pain was crushing — characteristic of a heart attack (myocardial infarction).

Teresa reacted to this with the pragmatic response that this 'might be it'. She imagined that this would not be a bad way to go, tucked up in bed at home. She explained the situation to Agnes. They both agreed that this would be an appropriate time for Bill to die, and nice for him to die at home. But Bill was in pain, and certainly needed something powerful to relieve this.

Teresa phoned their GP, who agreed that their plan was reasonable. He said he'd come.

Twenty minutes later, Bill's pain seemed much worse. He was writhing in agony and was having trouble breathing. Teresa could hear bubbling in his chest and there was white froth on his lips. Teresa called the surgery again. The GP said he was trying to come as quickly as he could, but he had other crises to deal with. He suggested they call an ambulance.

The ambulance was there in five minutes. The crew treated Bill meticulously, following their heart-attack protocol. Then they loaded him into the ambulance and took him to hospital.

Teresa and Agnes followed by car. They weren't familiar with the hospital and it took them a while to find a carpark and get to the emergency department. By the time they arrived, a lot had happened. An ECG had confirmed that Bill had suffered a massive heart attack.

Unfortunately, Bill had lost consciousness on the way in, and the ambulance officer had inserted a breathing tube into Bill's trachea and put him on a mechanical ventilator. Bill had also suffered a number of cardiac arrests and had been shocked several times. The shocks had restarted his heart.

The doctors were discussing sending Bill straight to the Cardiac Theatre to try to 'open up' the blocked artery in his heart.

Teresa was aghast. She had simply wanted her father

to get medication to help his pain and distress — but now she felt that there was a manic process underway that she was unable to control.

Teresa shared her concern about what was happening, but was reassured by the doctors that everything that was being done needed to be done. She told them that it was Bill's wish to be kept comfortable without 'heroics'. She asked that the breathing tube be removed and that there be no further measures to treat his heart attack (except for good pain relief).

Teresa was a forceful lady who could clearly state her opinion and, in my experience, had never been shy to do so. She was generally right when she put her foot down.

The cardiologist responded by suggesting that maximal treatment be given for 24 hours to see if things settled, and then to stop if it didn't work. Teresa couldn't see the value in this. She said no.

Teresa felt that nobody was listening to her. She rang me for support (although we had worked together years earlier, she remembered me, and I remembered her when she called. She had been memorable, in a good way).

I listened and reassured her. Her decision seemed consistent with what she said her dad had wanted (about getting out before his dementia got too advanced). Her interpretation of her father's wishes was also supported by Agnes. There were no other close family, so it looked like there was family consensus.

The doctors bowed to the family's wishes.

Bill was taken off the breathing machine with enough medication to make sure he was perfectly comfortable.

Teresa felt that by calling the ambulance, she had let Bill down, depriving him of his wish to die at home.

Later, on reflection, she told me that she was shocked to find how forceful she had needed to be in order to 'stop the steamroller' of medical care. It worried her that it took all her power (as a very confident, very determined, highly experienced nurse) to stop the process. She wondered what chance there would be for an ordinary person who had less knowledge, less confidence, and a much less forceful personality.

Teresa's experience is not uncommon. It can be very difficult to stop the process of treatment escalation. Doctors and the system are primed to cure, to save, and to heal — to do the opposite is confronting and disconcerting for clinicians.

Stephanie's story

Stephanie was an active 83-year-old who loved her garden. She was supportive to her wide circle of friends. Her husband, Cyril, had died five years earlier.

Stephanie valued her independence and her role as matriarch of her family, of whom she was very proud. She also enjoyed a role as an inspiration to her friends (and she had many).

When she turned 85, Stephanie started to deteriorate.

She repeatedly told her family that she would rather be dead than be dependent on others, and be unable to do the things that she enjoyed. She said that being able to independently manage in her own home was particularly important to her.

She appointed her eldest daughter, Jessie, to make medical treatment decisions for her, should she ever become unable to do so. She explained to the rest of the family that she had appointed Jessie because she felt that Jessie would be most likely to make the decisions that she herself would make. Stephanie asked the family to respect her decision to appoint Jessie and to respect any treatment choice that Jessie might make.

Just before Christmas, Stephanie fell from a chair she was standing on. She was trying to put things on the top shelf of a cupboard. Jessie called in and found Stephanie unconscious on the floor.

In hospital, it quickly became clear that Stephanie had suffered a major head injury and had broken her neck. There was evidence of spinal cord injury. It was clear that she would never walk again, nor have voluntarily control of her bladder or bowel function.

The situation was discussed with the family. The doctor later told me that she had explained that there could be some recovery from the head injury, but that the severity of the spinal injury meant that this could not be expected to recover. While rehabilitation and adaptation to life in a wheelchair would be possible, this would be difficult for an elderly person.

Answering questions from the family, she had explained that she felt that there was no prospect that Stephanie could manage independently in her own home.

There was a family discussion. This focused on what Stephanie would want, rather than what the family wanted. They tried not to be swayed by their wish not to lose Stephanie, whom they clearly loved.

When they had finished, Jessie went back to see the doctor. She explained that the family felt that Stephanie would not want treatment to prolong her life.

Jessie said that as the appointed agent, she wished this decision to be respected by the medical staff. The doctor acknowledged the decision.

Stephanie was admitted under the palliative care team, who made it their priority to keep Stephanie comfortable. She died peacefully four days later, without regaining consciousness.

The things that contribute to a good death have been the subject of quite extensive research and discussion. There seem to be some common themes, which include the following: being at home (or as close to this sort of environment as is practically possible); dying reasonably quickly without pain or suffering; having family present, and having the opportunity to say goodbye; dealing with unfinished emotional business (e.g., saying sorry, and hearing others say sorry); leaving affairs in good order. Other themes involve more personal and poetic sorts of wishes: to be in a favourite place, to have a particular person present, to have particular music playing — things like that.

Modern medicine, with its institutions and technology, regularly orchestrates a death that violates all of these aspirations. It's a paradox. There is a huge gulf between what we say we want and what actually happens.

The next consideration is 'permission'. It can be so liberating when those who are dying are able to assure their family that 'it's all right to let me go' — relieving them of the concern that doing nothing means that they don't care or don't love enough. This is permission for them to accept, permission that families crave.

It works the other way round, too. It provides great relief to dying patients when their family assures them that it is not necessary to endure or to suffer 'for the family'.

Permission is so important, but this need is rarely appreciated. Hannah understood. I'd like to share her story with you:

Hannah's story

Over many years, I cared for a plucky little girl with cystic fibrosis. Her name was Hannah. Hers was a particularly severe case. We saw a lot of each other in the hospital, much more than Hannah would have wanted.

Hannah finally hit the wall in her early teens. There was no magic solution. Her lungs were wrecked.

For a variety of reasons, transplantation wasn't a possibility.

Hannah's family was rough and tough. Her father was unemployed. But they were lovely, caring, reliable parents. Neither said much — they just went on with things and made the best of it.

Lying in her hospital bed, Hannah looked so tiny, so emaciated, and was so breathless.

Amazingly, she rallied. She told her mum and dad that she knew how much they loved her. She told them that she loved them, too.

She told them that it was OK . They hugged her and told her that it was fine if it was time for her to go.

It was.

As a doctor, I see a lot of emotion and think that I generally cope pretty well. But on this occasion, I made a quiet apology and left. They didn't need me. I closed my office door and cried. Hannah was very brave and very special.

Often the greatest wisdom comes from the most unexpected places.

Frequently, patients endure not because it is what they want, but they do so 'for the family'.

Often, we hear families telling dying relatives that they

'mustn't go', that they 'can't leave'. In these situations, there's no permission to go — quite the opposite.

Guilt is another big consideration. Family members can be left with a lot of guilt when responsibility for decision-making is put onto them. This feeling can easily prevent decisions to step back from ineffective or unwanted treatment.

One devoted mother expressed this concern very clearly when she observed: 'If I say "let him go", I know it is best for him, but it also seems as if I want it to happen. Like I want him to die and I don't care. I could never say "let him go" because I can never accept the other things.'

Another problem is that substitute decision-makers can often make decisions that satisfy their own needs rather than addressing the wishes of the patient for whom they are choosing.

Statements such as 'I know Mum would never want this, but I can't let her go' or 'He wouldn't want it, but we have to give him a chance' suggest that the substitute's needs are driving the decision (and they are not representing the person properly).

Comments such as this should provoke further discussion to refocus on the interests and wishes of the patient, rather than what the family (or others) want. There are some useful questions to employ here, such as, 'What do you think he would want?' and 'What do you think he would say if he were sitting here with us now?'

These types of questions often result in a surprisingly

clear expression of the person's wishes. It nicely highlights the personality of the person and 'brings them into the room'.

CHAPTER 4

How to avoid getting what you don't want

Because everyone is so keen to keep you alive, it is necessary to provide lots of clear, unambiguous guidance so that everyone can be quite certain that if they *do* strive to keep you alive, it would be quite wrong (and you would not be pleased).

This is a big task — a bigger one that most people appreciate.

Of course, if you fear that others might 'let you go' out of misguided kindness, then you should also make this clear, so they know to keep going without worrying, too.

There are some important things to do to help ensure that wishes are followed.

Doctors, and the medical system, work on the assumption that anyone who does not have a plan wants everything possible done to try to save them.

This assumption is wrong, but the system won't change.

It is our personal responsibility to set our own limits. It's important and necessary. Refusing to set limits often has consequences.

Alice's story

A while ago, I appeared on a panel exploring the topic of 'Not-for-Resuscitation'. The topic generated some lively debate. The organisers had invited Alice, a feisty elderly lady, to make the case against never 'giving in' by declining life-saving treatment.

She was a likeable, larger-than-life character, who was in her late 80s. She explained her optimistic view of life, and how she had always rebelled against expectations and authority.

She told us that she did her housework 'naked', and revelled in the idea that this might shock. When it came to 'Not-for-Resuscitation', she said that she was an optimist, and proudly asserted that if anyone tried to talk to her about not being resuscitated she'd certainly tell him to 'piss off'.

She was a personality. Feedback was overwhelmingly admiring. The audience liked Alice's view that optimism was a great way to deal with concern about the future. They agreed that planning, or setting limits, was pessimistic.

I liked Alice and I liked her performance, but I worried about her message.

I know from experience that every day, doctors have
to make choices (with families) about what to do in the
best interest of people who are so ill that they can't say
what they'd want.

When someone refuses to talk about limits, we have to
assume that they'd want us to do 'whatever it takes' to save
them, and act accordingly.

Would this really be what Alice would want, though?
Let's imagine Alice had a huge stroke the next week (she was
certainly at an age where these things happen). Let's say this
stroke destroyed her ability to do housework (and certainly
to do it naked!), removed all possibility of her staying in
her own home, and stopped her being able to communicate
meaningfully.

Would Alice want us to do everything possible to save
her (including resuscitation)? I saw clues that she may not
want this. Her ability to express herself through flamboyant,
contrary behaviour seemed to be an important aspect of
who she was. Her independence and outrageousness seemed
important to her. I found it difficult to believe that she
would be at ease in a nursing home; on the contrary, I think
she'd fight everything and hate every moment.

But this is conjecture — we can't know with enough
certainty. Without clear guidance (from Alice) to 'piss off',
I don't think anyone would feel confident to do less than
everything possible to save her. Hopefully, this would be

exactly what she *would* want.

It was a while ago now. I often wonder what happened to Alice. I wonder if there was a time when difficult decisions needed to be made. I hope that her refusal to plan didn't turn out badly for her.

The desire to understand what someone wants (and doesn't want) is neither inherently bad nor is it motivated by badness. It is an important part of having respect for individuals, and an important initiative to try to ensure that all treatment is really wanted.

Many people believe that 'when the time comes', their family and doctor will 'know what to do'. This seems especially true of older people who seem particularly trusting. Unfortunately, such confidence is generally unfounded.

Phoebe's story

Phoebe wasn't a patient of mine but of one of my colleagues, Mike, who works (almost on his own) in a remote country town. He told me this story.

Phoebe was one of his older patients. She lived alone in a small unit in town, having retired from running the post office. She was well liked locally. She had no known family.

Phoebe was generally well, and only saw Mike occasionally for little things.

Phoebe was brought to the town's hospital with sudden massive bleeding from her lower bowel. When

Mike saw her, blood was literally pouring from her bottom, her blood pressure was un-recordable, and she was semi-conscious. (This sort of massive bleeding is quite commonly in the elderly.)

Mike started fluid resuscitation and organised urgent transfer to the larger hospital where I work, so that the source of the bleeding could be identified and could hopefully be controlled (it usually can be).

While he was still on the phone making arrangements, Phoebe woke up (Mike's treatment had restored her blood pressure). She made it very clear that she did not want to be sent away and didn't want anything done. She seemed entirely lucid, calling him 'chook', as she always did. She confirmed that she perfectly understood the consequences and she didn't care. She wasn't consenting to the transfer.

Mike cancelled everything.

Phoebe expressed some surprise that Mike didn't realise that she'd never want to 'get sent away'. She trusted Mike to 'do the right thing' if he couldn't sort her out.

Mike kept Phoebe in their hospital. The bleeding stopped (on its own) and Phoebe survived. She was never interested in investigating the cause of the bleeding. It didn't happen again, and Phoebe lived for several more years.

Mike expressed frustration because, as he said, he wasn't psychic, and she hadn't given him any clue about these wishes. Phoebe had never talked to him about dying, and he had never raised it with her. It was a turning point for him. He now has what he calls 'what if' conversations with his patients on a regular basis.

In many cases, people only leave general comments about wishes that can be very hard to interpret. For instance, would it be reasonable to assume that a patient would not accept treatment after a stroke if they had previously commented 'I would never want to be like that!' when observing the life of someone severely disabled after a stroke? Could this be regarded as a considered statement of wishes? Or should it be rejected as an inappropriate, ill-considered, insensitive, 'throwaway' remark?

In real life, such 'social' comments are often all that we have to go on. It is on such evidence that family and doctors try to determine wishes.

How should we react when a person has repeatedly stated, over a number of weeks or months, that they 'can't go on'? Is it reasonable to assume that they would have no desire for life-sustaining treatment? Or should we assume that 'can't go on' means 'can't go on like this', and that this person might actually want treatment to change the way things are? Is this evidence of refusal or simply a comment that expresses frustration?

Similarly, how should a request for 'No unnecessary life support' be interpreted where a patient is failing to improve on prolonged life support? In this situation, life support is clearly *necessary* to maintain life (so is not 'unnecessary'), but is unlikely to restore health. 'Necessary' clearly needs more explanation.

It's just the same for 'heroic'. What would this person regard as heroic?

It is easy to see how these statements might be interpreted quite differently by various family members or by different doctors. Different interpretations feed conflict and confusion.

In addition to the statements themselves being ambiguous, it is not uncommon to find that a person will have said different things, at different times, to different people. Sometimes, we say conflicting things to people, often trying to be more positive to those who seem most distressed.

It is very important to be aware that what we say and what we write down *really does matter*.

Being vague or contradictory is likely to result in treatment that is unwanted or could mean missing out on treatment that you would want.

It is best to try to avoid making a plan that looks like an 'each-way bet'. It's tempting to try, because most of us like to keep our options open. We want to live as long as we can (providing our life has quality), and we don't want to be denied a chance to live — but we also don't want to live badly or suffer horribly. So we 'sort of' express concerns, but leave enough ambiguity to ensure we won't be denied treatment that could work. Ambiguity risks doctors 'half trying', which can be bad as it generally results in failure — bad failure, because the opportunity for focus on comfort, dignity, and humanity will have been compromised by the need to try (a bit) to cure.

However, it is possible to communicate an 'each-way bet' unambiguously by making it clear that simple treatments that are not uncomfortable are wanted (leaving open the chance to be saved), while excluding more unpleasant treatments that are less likely to work by expressing a desire that failure of simple treatments should not lead to an escalation to these.

We also know that people who say that they would *never, ever* accept something often change their mind in a crisis when they are faced with a real decision. Doctors know this and expect people to accept things they have previously rejected.

A lot of people express a wish not to be kept alive in situations where they would be significantly incapacitated. However, we know from experience that people who become disabled show a remarkable ability to adapt and accept. This makes it difficult to take seriously a 'line in the sand' (the minimum quality of life that a person is willing to accept) that has been expressed when someone is well.

If we were to accept this argument, then we would have to reject *all* requests to forgo treatment. This would cause huge distress and great outrage for those who really do want to avoid a complicated end, and who expect their wishes to be respected. We are left in that difficult situation where we have a flawed option that is less flawed than the alternative.

If you are sure about what you don't want, then it is important to ask that your wishes be respected and that others not speculate about any future change of mind.

Where plans have worked well (those cases where nobody had any doubt at all that it was right to follow the plan), there is clear agreement by everyone involved that the wishes are clear, firm, and unswerving.

Advance directives often give some indication of wishes, but they are often not specific enough, or written recently enough, to provide the degree of confidence that doctors and family need to support a decision to withhold treatment.

This point is well demonstrated by considering the situation of a person who has tattooed 'Not for CPR' across their chest. This might seem to be the clearest advance directive possible, indicating that the person really does not want resuscitation.

However, when asked to discuss this case, doctors and nurses readily identify concerns: Could this person have changed their mind, but have been unable to remove the tattoo? (Tattoos are very hard to get off.) Were they properly informed of the current chances of successful resuscitation? Does the tattoo mean they want to exclude resuscitation in *all* circumstances, even if there is a 100 per cent chance of success?

And finally, of course, to tattoo this on your chest is a rather extreme act. There may be doubt about the sanity and competence of a person who goes this far.

Listening to this concern, it doesn't take long to appreciate how difficult it is to create a directive that provides the degree of certainly that doctors and family members require to feel confident to act on it.

Knowing a person's values, how they think, and what gives their life meaning (including things that they would really want to avoid) can support confident medical decision-making.

Let me share an example that happened to me recently:

Madeleine's story

Madeleine was, and still is, an elderly nurse. I came to know her because of a shared interest in a community group where she is a major force.

Madeleine's identity was intimately involved in caring for others in need.

Madeleine knew of my interest in planning and had told me she had completed an advance care plan in which she said that she would not want CPR.

I provide emergency cover on occasional weekends at a small hospital in the country town where Madeleine lives (I do it primarily so that the regular GP gets a chance to get away, but it is also very different from my regular job and I enjoy the variety).

It was on one of these weekends that Madeleine was brought in by ambulance. She had severe chest pain, looked ashen, and was sweating profusely.

An ECG promptly revealed that Madeleine was having an acute heart attack — and it looked to be a big one. We quickly administered the appropriate cocktail of clot-busting treatment and everything improved (suggesting that the treatment was working and that blood was again starting to flow down the blocked artery to supply her heart muscle).

As Madeleine improved, her greatest concern, for which she repeatedly apologised, was that she was out in company wearing her old gardening stockings (she had been gardening when she became unwell). She was horrified that she was not dressed more appropriately in public! The stockings looked fine to me, but it mattered to Madeleine.

The next events were rather predictable.

When blood flow is returned to heart muscle that has been deprived of oxygen, the muscle is saved from dying — but it often becomes irritable. This irritability can set off ventricular fibrillation (where the heart muscle just quivers rather than properly contracting, and the heart stops pumping blood). The irritability settles down over a number of hours, but it is a real risk soon after blood flow is restored. Ventricular fibrillation, otherwise called a cardiac arrest, is something that requires urgent defibrillation (resuscitation) to restore an effective heart rhythm — or the person will die. This was what Madeleine had refused in her plan.

Madeleine suddenly stopped talking about her stockings, rolled up her eyes, and became unconscious. The monitor showed ventricular fibrillation. An instant decision needed to be made.

On one hand, there was a strong argument to respect Madeleine's autonomy, her undoubted right to have her documented wishes respected — and she had a clearly expressed wish not to be resuscitated. It was written down, signed, and witnessed (though I wasn't involved in creating it and had not discussed it with her).

On the other hand, it was possible to consider the actual clinical situation and the likely outcome of treatment, and to try to match this information with Madeleine's values.

I was witnessing her arrest, and it was only seconds since her heart had stopped. There would be no significant heart or brain damage if we restarted her heart quickly. I also knew that this sort of ventricular fibrillation that occurs after clot-busting treatment is generally easy to treat and almost always results in a full recovery. I would also be treating a predictable side effect of an expensive treatment that had already been started, so in a way it could be considered to be part of that treatment.

This was an unusual situation, because I knew more about Madeleine than is the case for most patients I treat.

I speculated that Madeleine's decision to refuse

resuscitation was most likely based on a determination not to get into a situation where she would need to be cared for. Her life narrative revolved around caring for others. Being cared for didn't fit with how she saw her life. I had tried to get Madeleine to accept being cared for previously when she had been sick, and it had been a disaster. She proved to be a terrible patient. Without this narrative of caring for others, it was likely that her life might lose important meaning, from her perspective. Dignity also seemed to be important to Madeleine; in this context, her worry about the gardening stockings was completely in character.

I was sure that if we resuscitated Madeleine she would make a full recovery, and the things that were likely to be the basis of her refusal of resuscitation (the risk of dependency and indignity) were extremely unlikely. This had to be balanced with the problem of ignoring a clear instruction, which would disrespect Madeleine's right to make her own decision, even a decisions that I (or others) might disagree with.

This had to be a quick decision. Delay would result in brain damage.

I opted to resuscitate. One shock worked. The whole process of thought and action probably took only a few seconds.

Madeleine quickly regained consciousness and, not realising what had happened, was straight back to apologising about her stockings. She was transferred safely to a major hospital that had a cardiac intervention service, where she had a stent quickly and effectively placed into the diseased artery. Madeleine was home, fixed, a few days later.

As Madeleine had a clear directive against CPR, I needed to talk to her about what had happened. I paid her a visit soon after she got home.

She provided tea, chocolate biscuits, and cake on her best china.

I explained how her heart had stopped and how we had restarted it. She asked if that would have been 'resuscitation', and I confirmed that it was. She was instantly indignant, claiming that her directive had been 'ignored'. This was totally in character; Madeleine is feisty, and being respected is very important to her.

She told me that she had seen some very poor outcomes after resuscitation in others, and this was something she was very worried about — something she was determined to avoid by never letting herself be resuscitated.

I told her how I had tried to interpret her directive in the context of what I knew of her values and priorities. I asked if she felt this was a fair thing for me to have done. She did. I asked her how she would have felt if I had followed her instruction and had 'let her go'. She assured me that that would have been fine because, as she put it, 'you'd only be doing what I asked you to do'.

We revised her directive to include more explanation of what she really wanted to avoid. It is now years since that memorable Saturday. Madeleine remains very well. I see her often, and she is just as active as ever as she cares for everyone.

She still has her plan.

In this case, knowledge of values proved a more convincing and useful basis for decision-making than was the instruction in the written directive.

Madeleine hadn't appointed anyone to be a substitute decision-maker for her, but this can be one way to ensure that values (and fears) are considered in decision-making.

An appointed substitute is able to evaluate the circumstances of the specific clinical event, present the values of the person, and engage in a dialogue with doctors — effectively sharing the decision-making.

This sort of process is close to what patients themselves do when making decisions. Few of us come into a medical situation with a pre-existing decision set in concrete; most of us want to discuss options and to have our values, wishes, and fears considered.

Some doctors reject the validity of patient-selected substitute or family decision-making. However, such rejection relies on the premise that the doctor is a better end-of-life decision-maker than family or appointed substitutes. Against this argument is evidence that doctors themselves often wrongly predict patient's desires regarding end-of-life treatment.

It is really important that someone who is asked to act as a substitute is up to the task, and appreciates how difficult this task is likely to be. Passing responsibility to someone who finds decision-making difficult is not wise (because you may well not get what you want), and is unfair to the person appointed (because they are liable to end up damaged by the process).

We all procrastinate, but it is important not to leave planning until it is too late. A small, but revealing, survey of elderly, chronically ill housebound patients found that most chose to avoid planning. They considered that end-of-life matters were in the hands of God, and not their responsibility!

Ninety-five per cent were reluctant to think about, discuss, or plan for serious future illness. This was very unfortunate, as life-threatening deterioration was almost certain for this group of patients — and likely in the very near future. Rather than planning, they described a 'one day at a time' attitude, a 'what will be, will be' approach to life, preferring to 'cross that bridge' when they got to it.

Those who had an advance directive intended it to apply *only* when death was both very near and absolutely certain. They didn't intend the plan to apply in an acute, life-threatening medical situation where death was probable but not certain. They provided no guidance for this, even though, for them, a life-threatening medical emergency was highly likely.

These observations are important because they question

the ability of those who are very sick and elderly to plan — and it is this group for whom it is most urgent and important. This challenges the assumption that we should delay thinking about severe illness until death is imminent.

Thinking about a plan when we are still fit and well means we can think clearly about the issues, without undue pressure or emotion, and have plenty of time to think and discuss everything. Planning well in advance of something happening is not that alien a concept for us — we do it when we make a will or take out insurance.

Planning is easier if we think about values (what matters to us) rather than thinking about death and dying (which are difficult). Our values define us; they make us who we are. Values form the basis of *how* we think about things, and they predict things about how we will react.

We can hold a variety of different values at the same time, some of which may conflict with others. Making decisions often involves sorting out how our values apply to the issues under consideration.

Many of us have some values that we hold more strongly than others. These are things we feel that we would never overrule. These 'fundamental' values are important because they are strong and relatively resistant to change.

Someone who reaffirms similar values in various situations (when the context is changed) or someone who repeatedly, and confidently, expresses the same view is likely to hold this value reasonably strongly.

When a value 'fits' with the personality, identity, or

narrative of an individual, it adds confidence to the reliability of the expressed value. For example, a view supporting the sanctity of life might 'fit' with the identity and narrative of someone who also expressed strong religious conviction. Alternatively, a choice based on respect for personal autonomy might 'fit' with someone who is also a strong supporter of progressive social causes.

Exploring values, fears, and wishes may identify factors that are critical for an individual: those things that they hold strongly, things that underpin their decisions. Identifying which factors are most critical, and how they interact, is inevitably subjective and unique to each situation — but with listening and consideration they can often resolve to reveal a credible solution.

Solving this dilemma is easier if we can understand what is meant by values. Values include beliefs about what is desirable or positive, together with an understanding of what is considered to be negative or futile.

Values are deep-felt, long-established, and unchanging attitudes that explain how and why different realities matter to us as individuals.

As well as positive values, we have 'disvalues' — things we consider undesirable, harmful, or unworthy. They identify realities that we dislike and would wish to avoid.

Preferences naturally flow from values — for example, 'I place a high value on privacy (value), so I detest the thought of unknown strangers wiping my bottom (preference) and I would not accept this.'

Values and personality seem to be rather stable over adulthood, while preferences may vary, depending on circumstances.

Obtaining an idea of the strength with which each value is held and the context in which it may apply (in the view of the individual concerned) provides information about how a person *thinks*, and how the individual is likely to respond to trade-offs — will they drop one value in favour of another? Trade-offs occur in most complex decisions. In the context of medical treatment, these can include, for example, the person's attitude to pain-relief medication (located on a spectrum between minimising pain and maximising consciousness), and their attitude to safety (between being kept safe and having the freedom to take risks).

Considering values provides a basis for discussion and opens the way for a dialogue that can help us to predict and understand preferences. If we understand someone's values, it makes their wishes easier to respect, especially when they 'fit' with values.

However, preferences can change, so this isn't an exact science. An interesting study, performed on a group of very elderly patients who were all considered to be cognitively intact and who were living in the community, explored this.

These patients had an average age of 88 (with a range from 84 to 100). Eighty per cent had previously indicated a preference for comfort care over life-extending care, and it was this group that the study looked at.

They were asked if they would reject a hypothetical

uncomfortable life-prolonging treatment that was offered to them over sticking with their previously expressed choice to opt for comfort (and death). Given the choice, 20 per cent accepted the life-extending treatment.

This study was conducted in America (which may be significant, because Americans appear to take a more positive attitude towards life support than do those in other countries).

The authors make the important point that the patients in their study may not have fully understand that their stated preference for 'comfort care' would exclude interventional treatment.

It is also likely that they may have been unaware of what the experience of the intervention would be and the poor chances of them returning home.

Interestingly, though the patients in the study were so elderly, only 12 per cent reported ever having discussed their wishes or goals with their doctor. Clearly, this is disappointing, but is similar to findings in other studies. It seems that doctors won't discuss end of life, even with an 88-year-old, leaving patients ill-informed, confused, and unsupported.

The authors of this study concluded that advance plans can't reliably predict treatment preferences. But I think, perhaps, they may have missed something important that might have been clarified with one more question: they could have asked those who had a change of mind, 'How would you feel if your family and doctor had chosen to follow your previous wish for comfort and had not offered the treatment?'

From my experience, I think that they would have acknowledged that the decision was difficult. They would not have expected others to be able to guess the answer that they came up with, and they would have accepted that respecting their previously expressed choice (for comfort care) was perfectly reasonable — even though this was not what they ended up choosing themselves.

To take things further, they could also have been asked: 'Would you be *angry* with them for declining treatment?' I doubt many would feel this way.

Looked at in this way, the original wishes would not be considered as unreliable but instead would provide useful guidance. And we shouldn't forget that the study also showed that three out of four of the elderly patients *did* stick with their original decision to forgo life-prolonging treatment in favour of comfort care.

Worry about the stability of a person's choices gives more reason to try to better understand the basis of 'how' they think by exploring their values, wishes, and fears. Ongoing discussion can identify the strength of the views, which gives a sense of how likely these are to change.

Despite all this, we know that wishes can change profoundly during the final stages of life. This observation is often used as an argument to support ignoring previously expressed wishes.

Before accepting such a sweeping assessment, we should think a bit about what is happening in these final stages.

As death becomes 'real', health professionals and

families often feel increasingly motivated to act and try to 'do something', while the patient may be pragmatic and accepting.

Dying people are placed in a situation where they are left to wage a lonely battle of ideas between an advocacy for intervention from just about everyone they come in contact with (family, doctors, friends) and a pragmatic acceptance that nobody else seems willing to respect.

Faced with this, it can be little surprise that choices oscillate wildly. Such pressure at this vulnerable time seems unfair, unsettling, and unkind.

There is a strong argument that a patient's prior wishes should be taken seriously, and that they should be supported to maintain these wishes through crisis.

The suggestion that prior (well-considered) wishes should carry more weight than a later decision made in crisis (often with more emotion and less thought) is supported by the work of the psychologist Daniel Kanneman. He suggests that choices made as a result of thought are more reliable, more stable, and 'safer' than decisions made under stress, which are often driven by emotion. Daniel Kanneman received a Nobel Prize for his work on decision-making, so it is probably reasonable to take him fairly seriously. But in practice, thoughtful, considered advance decisions are routinely overlooked in favour of decisions that are made in crisis, under conditions of great stress, and which are often subject to overwhelming external pressure.

To get a better understanding of what people value

towards the end of life, our research group conducted a study in collaboration with the Centre for the Study of Choice. These are academic experts who try to understand human decision-making.

Human choice is fascinating. It is rarely entirely logical. We want everything good and nothing bad, and we want it all at once; real choices only become clear when we are forced to make trade-offs. This becomes particularly important when investigating wishes about something really unattractive, like death.

We studied 1166 adults aged over 55, who were resident in Australia, using a proven experimental design (Best–Worst Scoring) with the Centre for the Study of Choice. We examined the participants' enthusiasm for medical treatment in hypothetical situations of poor health.

We also provided them with a series of scenarios where the intensity of treatment increased as the likely benefit decreased (to see how far they would want to go). Analysis of our results revealed three distinct groups (with a fourth group where wishes could not be defined).

The first group were strongly opposed to any intervention to prolong life in poor health or poor quality. This group had a particular aversion to being kept alive with cognitive impairment. They comprised 61 per cent of respondents aged over 75 and 42 per cent of those aged less than 75. This group gave clear positive scores (agreement) to statements that began 'I would rather die than …' They gave a strongly negative score to the statement 'All human life is sacred.'

The second group favoured medical intervention, no matter what the chances of success and/or the degree of impairment. They comprised 7 per cent of respondents aged over 75 and 6 per cent of those aged less than 75. For this group, there was strongest agreement to the statement 'All human life is sacred', while the three statements that included the words 'I would rather die than ...' were the least popular.

A third group was mildly 'anti-treatment', but wanted to retain treatment options and were willing to trade off aspects of treatment and outcomes. This group took 'each decision on its merits'. They reacted negatively to the 'I would rather die than ...' statements, but much less powerfully than was the case for the second group. They comprised the remaining 32 per cent of respondents aged over 75 and 33 per cent of those aged less than 75.

The remaining 19 per cent of those aged less than 75 (group four) had no discernible pattern of preferences. Either their ideas were all over the place and defied analysis, or they didn't take the survey seriously and just entered random answers. We couldn't discern anything from this group, and didn't include their answers in any further analysis.

The results suggested to us that the majority of older Australians are concerned about quality at the end of their lives (particularly as it applies to mental functioning), with only a small minority (6–7 per cent) wanting to 'extend life at all costs'. It is probably reasonable to conclude that attitudes would be broadly similar in other countries.

This observation is important because it is inconsistent with the current default position of families, doctors, and of society as a whole — to try to extend life whenever possible, even where predicted outcomes are poor.

Ivan's story

It didn't take long for us to appreciate that Ivan was one of that 7 per cent for whom living is the number one priority. He seemed willing to do everything to stay alive. I regularly see patients like Ivan and they generally get every possible treatment, but Ivan was a memorable example.

Ivan had widespread prostate cancer. He had had treatment for his cancer, but, because of side effects, it had been stopped. New lesions on his scans suggested that the chemotherapy he had received hadn't been all that effective. The cancer was causing a lot of bone pain, for which his palliative-care doctor was prescribing large doses of strong opiate pain relief.

Before coming to hospital, Ivan was managing at home with help from his wife and two daughters (both of whom had given up work to care for him), but there had been some concern that it was getting too much. Ivan was a big man, who now needed help to get out of bed and was becoming unsteady on his feet.

Ivan had appointed his younger daughter, Natalia, as his substitute medical decision-maker. Natalia had worked as a nurse, though not for some years, but Ivan felt she would be the best choice because she understood 'how the medical system works' and was close to him.

I first met Ivan after he was rushed to hospital with terrible pain in his abdomen. The emergency department had already organised a scan, which showed clear evidence that most of Ivan's bowel had lost its blood supply, and was dead. This can sometimes be a bit difficult to be sure about on scans, but in Ivan's case it was beyond doubt.

The emergency doctor and the on-call surgeon had already talked to the family, including Natalia. They were adamant that Ivan would want surgery (though Ivan was much too ill and confused to say so for himself). This was in the setting of a poor prognosis for his cancer, ongoing bone pain, evidence of struggling to stay at home, a near hopeless chance of surviving surgery to get home, and a predictably difficult, complicated journey after surgery if he were to survive it.

The surgeon wasn't at all keen to operate and asked us to add more detail about the expected intensive-care experience.

As we talked, the family conveyed a very clear and consistent narrative — Ivan would certainly want surgery, he didn't want to die, and would want to do whatever necessary to avoid dying. The risks meant nothing to him.

Furthermore, they saw his cancer in an unusual way — in their minds, Ivan had stopped treatment because his cancer was under such good control ('remission'), and because he hadn't felt that the side effects were 'worth it' when the treatment wasn't really necessary anyway.

Ivan got his operation, and the dead half of his bowel was removed. He required significant life support for weeks after his operation. This involved mechanical ventilation, and some days of dialysis. But slowly, amazingly, he improved and gradually got off the life support.

As soon as he properly woke up, Ivan confirmed that Natalia's decision (to ask the surgeons to operate) was exactly what he would have wanted. He also confirmed their story about how he saw his cancer.

As we got to know him better, it became obvious that this all fitted with his attitude and personality. Natalia had done an excellent job of communicating his approach and wishes.

Despite coming off life support, Ivan remained very ill and looked uncomfortable most of the time (despite being given generous doses of pain relief), but it didn't seem to upset him — it just wasn't that important. Every time we asked how he was doing, he would simply say 'better than the alternative' or 'still alive'. He seemed to enjoy being contrary.

After eight weeks in hospital, Ivan was transferred to a hospice. I spoke with him just before he left. He had no regrets and was happy to be alive.

It takes all sorts. Most of us would never want to go through what Ivan endured, seemingly for nothing. But then, we're not Ivan. It was Ivan's choice, and understanding values helped us to understand Ivan and what he wanted.

Most people find considering their 'values' to be much easier and more acceptable than having to decide about specific treatments in particular circumstances. Most of us don't mind sharing those things that we care about, things that make us 'who we are'. Indeed, most of us are flattered when others try to understand us!

Another advantage of considering values is that, as values reflect 'who we are', this is something that is quite fixed. 'Who we are' tends not to change too much as we go through life.

My dad had the same political views throughout his life, strong views about same-sex marriage, views about war, and views about just about everything else. I didn't agree with many of his opinions, but I respected his right to his beliefs, and, to be fair, he didn't tend to speak of them with strangers! These views never changed a jot. Just before he died (at 89), he wistfully told me that he was surprised to discover that the way he felt was just the same as he did when he was 20. He thought it would be different, but it wasn't.

When I meet old friends and family, they seem very much the same as when I met them last. Those things that made them 'who they were' before remain the same. These values don't tend to change over time, so are something we can reasonably consider well in advance.

As the research processes for ranking values are quite time consuming (for those doing the survey, that is) we devised a simpler tool that we called 'What Matters Most'.

'What Matters Most' invited people to identify the importance of just four attributes — 'maintaining dignity', 'avoiding pain and suffering', 'living as long as possible', and 'remaining independent'. Each was ranked on a five-point scale from 'not at all important' to 'vitally important'.

We then went on to look at the same thing a little differently. We asked them to identify which one of the four choices they would want their doctor to make the *number one priority* to guide their treatment.

We wondered if people might be more likely to choose 'living as long as possible' as the priority for their doctor, as a precaution to avoid any risk that they might miss out on a life-saving treatment.

So, what did we find?

Maintaining dignity, avoiding pain and suffering, and remaining independent were important for most people, with more than 90 per cent rating these as 'vitally important' or 'somewhat important'.

On the other hand 'living as long as possible' was not felt to be so important — 30–35 per cent rated it as 'not very important' or 'not important at all'.

When they were asked to select the one thing that they would want their doctor to make the priority, the message was even clearer: only 3 per cent nominated living as long as possible, and the other priorities were pretty evenly popular with maintaining dignity at 28 per cent, avoiding pain and suffering at 44 per cent, and remaining independent at 25 per cent.

These results certainly came as a bit of a shock to us, but the results were clear. Once again, the same message comes through, but this time even more clearly: living as long as possible is just not the number one priority — other things matter more. It is obvious that we need to consider those other things as we make treatment decisions.

So there we were. We knew values mattered, but we also knew that many people find it difficult to sort out what they really think (often holding contradictory wishes at the same time), and often don't know what to think about.

It seemed that there needed to be something clever to help people sort out what they think about the things that are important for decision-making.

First, we considered the sort of values that we felt people needed to think about, which aren't necessarily those that people naturally consider.

We considered the different concepts that people raise when they are confronted by difficult treatment decisions towards the end of life. During years of medical practice, we have heard thousands of these.

From these, we constructed a list of values. These were then separated into pro-interventional and non-interventional concepts (or attitudes). Here is what we came up with:

NON-INTERVENTIONAL ATTITUDES

Attitude to life	completed life, 'ready to go'
Attitude to death	death is inevitable / natural prepared and accepting
Burden of disease	intolerant of disability/suffering
Burden of treatment	concerned about prolonged, invasive treatment
Confidence in science	medical science has limits ('we all die')
Outcome	quality is essential
When odds are poor	influenced by large chance of loss
Dignity	going on too long is undignified
Control	need to control the process
Outlook	fear of future
Burden	antipathy to 'being a burden'
Religious obligation	no religious imperative
Family duty	autonomous choice

INTERVENTIONAL ATTITUDES

Attitude to life	uncompleted life, lots yet to do
Attitude to death	death is avoidable fearful and unprepared
Burden of disease	willing to accept disability/suffering
Burden of treatment	reassured by availability of treatment
Confidence in science	anything can be cured if you try enough
Outcome	being alive is most important
When odds are poor	attracted to a small chance of gain

135

Dignity	human dignity enhanced by struggle
Control	fatalistic, accepting
Outlook	optimism for future (or denial)
Burden	being cared for is 'my right'
Religious obligation	religious belief mandates fight for life
Family duty	required to stay alive for family

We ended up with 60 statements, based on these concepts. Many addressed similar concepts, but in slightly different ways. For instance, while one statement says 'doing whatever it takes' (which sounds rather brave), another talks of 'needing to go the distance' which sounds rather more reasonable and expected. Both of these statements address the concept of willingness to accept treatment, but from slightly different perspectives.

Where someone agrees with both of these statements ('doing whatever it takes' and 'needing to go the distance'), we might conclude that this person has a tendency to accept treatment. On the other hand, someone who rejects both statements probably wouldn't want to accept high-risk burdensome treatment. If they agree with the first statement but reject the second, this may not be something they have strong views about or feel very confident about expressing an opinion on. We are expected to have fixed views, but in reality it is not unusual to 'sit on the fence'. The way survey questions are constructed is often designed to make us choose in a particular way, but a slightly different question can easily elicit a very different answer.

The concept might be easier to convey with an example that has nothing to do with end-of-life decision-making.

In any debate about same-sex marriage, the question may sometimes be framed around 'marriage equality'. This focuses on equality — surely something everyone would be inclined to support. When rephrased to 'same-sex marriage', the issue is likely to be interpreted differently, with the focus on the fact that a marriage may occur between two people of the same sex, contrasting with the 'traditional' model of marriage.

It is likely that fewer people would agree with the second statement than the first (which is why the way questions are presented is so important) — *but* if someone readily agrees with both statements, then we can be reasonably confident about their position, more so than if we knew their answer to just one of these statements. Obviously, the opposite would also apply: we could be more confident about someone's attitude if they disagreed with both statements (particularly if they strongly disagreed). We would have an even better understanding of where they stood if we were also to know their attitude to other concepts, such as 'marriage is a religious institution' and 'marriage is for the purpose of creating children'.

Using a range of statements that explore related, but different, concepts, we can get a good idea of how someone thinks. It easily identifies those who have views that are at the extreme end of the spectrum (those who agree with all of the statements, or disagree with all of them) but, most importantly, it also conveys how those in the middle think.

We can utilise the same concept when we consider end-of-life choices. Here, it is really important to understand nuanced 'middle ground' views. Few of us are so determined that we would reject *all* treatment under *all* circumstances or so naive as to want *every* possible treatment under *any* circumstance. Most of us take a middle position. We want our choices respected, so we need an efficient way to reliably convey how we feel.

Considering our personal attitude to a range of statements that address aspects of things such as suffering, hope, burden, independence, and dignity can provide important insights into how we individually feel and how we think. This is the approach we use in the 'MyValues' online program (www.myvalues.org.au). It's intended to help people identify and communicate their values in regard to future medical treatment (when the outlook isn't good). It creates a report of the things that are consistently and strongly reported. This can act as an advance care plan on its own, or it can supplement other documentation to make wishes clearer. It's free to use, and most people find it easy to do. It is available to everyone, wherever you live.

An example of the sort of report that it creates is shown on the next page.

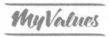

REPORT
16 NOVEMBER 2017

Mary Murphy

Strongly Held Views

- I would rather be dead than to have to go into a nursing home (long term)
- I would rather die than to need basic things such as feeding and toileting done for me (long term)
- Medical treatment has its limits. Keeping going too long is not appropriate when the odds of a good outcome are small
- I would prefer a treatment where the main aim was to ensure my comfort even if this treatment meant I would not live as long as a treatment that involved more discomfort

Analysis of thousands and thousands of responses to the various statements has revealed some interesting messages.

First, we are not all that consistent at a basic level. Lots of answers are very inconsistent. People can strongly agree (or disagree) with one statement, and then answer the complete opposite when the same concept is later presented in the opposite way — for instance agreeing with 'I would *never* want x' and only moments later agreeing with the statement 'I would want x if ...'

This observation is a strong argument against simplistic approaches to planning, where only a minimum of questions are asked, or worse, where a few tick-boxes are used to indicate choices.

Next, we can look at the answers that most people give. Do people 'want to live forever, whatever it takes'?

'Whatever it takes' is not supported by the data (at least as it applies to the thousands of people visiting the site). Eighty-eight per cent disagree (or strongly disagree) with the statement '"Never, never, ever give up" and "try, try, and try again" are a good summary of how I feel about my medical treatment.'

Even when this statement is presented in a way that makes agreement seem more reasonable — 'It is important to me to "go the distance", even when treatment is unpleasant, until it is absolutely clear that the treatment can never work' — 63 per cent of respondents disagree.

When life extension is associated with discomfort and forgoing more comfortable options — as reflected in the statement 'I would want treatment that aimed to extend my life as much as possible, even if this meant more pain and discomfort than alternative treatment aimed at keeping me comfortable' — it gets worse, and 81 per cent disagree.

Conversely, the concept that medicine has limits — 'Medical treatment has its limits. Keeping going too long is not appropriate when the odds of a good outcome are small' — resonates, with 92 per cent agreeing with this statement.

The prospect of ending up in a nursing home is not popular. In response to the statement 'I would rather be dead than have to go into a nursing home (long term)', 53 per cent stated a preference for death.

When the implication of high-level nursing-home care is less overt, and the statement focuses on things that people may consider undignified that often occur in nursing homes — 'I would rather die than need basic things such as feeding and toileting done for me (long term)' — this is even less popular, with 74 per cent suggesting that they would rather die.

There is one particular concept in the 'MyValues' survey that we felt might be particularly provocative, but revealing. It reflects something that commonly comes up in family discussion, but almost never gets raised in a conversation with doctors.

The statement was, '"Just push me off a cliff" and "take me to the back paddock and shoot me" are a good summary of how I feel, should I get into a bad state.'

Clearly, this is a metaphor, not something that anyone would realistically expect. Agreement with this statement indicates that the person looks positively on a decision to get death quickly over and done with when the time comes, rather than doing everything possible to fight it.

Among those who have completed the 'MyValues' survey, 56 per cent agree with this statement, while 7 per cent strongly disagree.

This statement proves to be a very good discriminator. The 7 per cent who strongly disagree with this statement generally give pro-intervention answers to most other questions, while those who like the idea (of being 'pushed off the cliff') tend to choose non-interventional responses across the rest of the statements.

There was more revelation to come from this statement. As an extension of the project, we translated the statements into a variety of languages. We used ethnic Arabic, Chinese, Vietnamese, Italian, and Greek translators for this task. None reported any difficulty with the concept of 'Just push me off a cliff ...', all reporting that this was a familiar concept in their culture.

When it came to translating, though, the Italian translator had some difficulty. He told us that he felt it would be morally wrong to suggest such a terrible thing (and he wouldn't do it). The translation he provided read: '"Gently roll me down a hill" and "take me out the back to lie in the long grass" are a good summary of how I feel, should I get into a bad state.'

We felt this was rather lovely, but that it completely missed the point! Maybe this says something interesting about Italian health care and communication (we got him to use our words).

There are two sorts of plan that are generally very easy for doctors and family to follow.

The first requests that absolutely everything possible be tried.

The second permits no treatment whatsoever in a life-threatening situation.

We see some plans like this, but few are this black-and-white. Most plans provide an intermediate instruction along the lines of 'I'd like an attempt to cure, but not too much', or provide a broad goal of care such as valuing 'quality of life'.

Unfortunately, these intermediate instructions prove almost impossible for others to interpret and implement. However, even these 'vague' plans do have some value.

'Make an attempt but not too much' turns out to be a reasonable predictor that the person will accept simple, non-aggressive intervention (e.g., antibiotic or intravenous fluid), but it fails to predict acceptance (or rejection) of more aggressive treatments.

On the other hand, a request for 'quality' reliably predicts rejection of the most extreme interventions (such as long-term mechanical ventilation), but it is not good at predicting whether a person would accept less-aggressive treatment (such as an operation) or a non-aggressive intervention (such as an antibiotic).

The problem arises because different people have very different attitudes about what constitutes 'quality' and what would be a 'reasonable' attempt to cure. Something that one person would regard as acceptable can easily turn out to be utterly unacceptable to the next, though they may have expressed exactly the same instruction.

Knowing that quality matters, or that an individual wouldn't want to go 'too far', is helpful, but it is not enough. It is also necessary to understand what constitutes quality of life for this particular individual or how burdensome they perceive different interventions would be, from their own particular perspective.

How a person treats uncertainty also needs to be understood. Would they only want to forgo treatment when the doctor is certain that it will not work (a very rare situation), or would they want to forgo treatment where there was a real risk of a poor outcome (for instance a 50 per cent chance)? These things can't be deduced from broad statements.

The next thing to recognise is that we can only be tough and clear about things that we are really confident about — we can't give clear instruction about things that we aren't certain about. Equally, we can't expect to have strong feelings about everything — there will always be things that we don't care that much about.

The important thing is to be *really clear* about those things that we do *feel strongly* about.

Avoiding ambiguity is vital. This is not the place for a 'maybe' or 'each-way bet'. Permitting ambiguity will simply ensure that there are no limits (which is unfortunate if it is your desire to set limits).

All this makes the process of completing advance care plans more complicated than most people appreciate.

Simply expressing wishes doesn't seem to be enough to stop them being ignored. Most doctors (and some families) believe that they have a duty to 'second guess' your wishes. In most cases, this means ignoring a wish to forgo treatment on the grounds that it's not possible to be sure that you have not changed your mind (or would not have a change of mind in the face of a real medical crisis).

Doctors frequently believe that everyone would expect them to overrule wishes that are, in their opinion, misguided. However the data shows the opposite: very few people want or expect this.

To stop wishes being overruled ('in your best interest'), it is advisable to state a desire, in the plan, that wishes not be overruled by the doctor.

The same advice applies to family decision-making. Few people want their family to override wishes, but countless times, I have heard families say, without a touch of irony, 'We know she wouldn't want it, but we want you to do it.' It is important to lock in your family to respecting your wishes. Telling them that they can demonstrate love by respecting your wishes can be an effective strategy. I realise it may seem a bit over the top to bring love into it — but they are going to find it very, very difficult not to buckle when the crisis comes and they need something really powerful to resist — and love can be very powerful. Simply asking for your wishes to be respected may be enough.

Plans need to be distributed as widely as possible — to family members (especially to those who are most difficult), to your GP, to your specialist, and to any hospital(s) that you attend. Sharing is important. The fact that you are willing to share expels the idea that this is something that you are hesitant about. If you don't share it with everyone, people can worry that you're keeping it hidden because you're unsure about it.

Finally, we come to the importance of the substitute decision-maker. Most families think that they have the duty, and the power, to make decisions about a relative's treatment. Many are very forceful (and not necessarily the most sensible ones, either). Families vary, but it is unusual for everyone to work collaboratively to agree on a well-thought-out decision about anything.

It is unusual for a great facilitator to emerge naturally (but it is nice when it happens).

Too commonly, a family dispute is sparked when difficult end-of-life treatment decisions have to be made. These decisions are often difficult and emotional. The stress easily opens existing divisions or brings out weaknesses. Positions are often taken to thwart opposing family factions, rather than to advance the interest of the patient.

The noisiest or the most forceful family members are often not the wisest or the most collaborative. Those selected by the family to be decision-makers are frequently the least appropriate (often being the most emotional or the most aggressive).

Recognising all this makes the prior selection and formal appointment of a substitute decision-maker ('agent') a really good idea. There are some important attributes of a good substitute decision-maker:

They need to recognise that they are acting for you, that they have a duty to understand your wishes and need to represent *your* interests (not their own).

Representing your interests is likely to involve following

any expressed wishes (to a greater or lesser extent). An agent should certainly be familiar with your wishes and should express respect for them.

Good substitute decision-makers need to be able to gain the respect of the other parties (doctors and family) — an aura of authority seems to help in this regard.

A good agent also needs to respect others. Asserting that they have all the authority, and everyone else's views are irrelevant, is unlikely to go down well. Ensuring that others — who also feel close and responsible — feel that they have been 'listened to' is very important (while at the same time limiting the influence of pushy, distant relatives). It is not always easy.

Substitute decision-makers need to be *good* decision-makers; appointing a poor decision-maker can be worse than doing nothing. Good decision-making means not making decisions with inadequate information, nor delaying indefinitely while awaiting information that might never come. It also means that they are able to live with their decision (whichever way the decision goes). The ability to rationalise that they did their best (with the information available) without later regrets is important. Some substitutes can experience years of unresolved guilt about a decision they have made.

Appointing someone who is likely to be damaged by the process is not only unfair on them, but they are also liable to make decisions that minimise their discomfort, rather than decisions that are best for you, or what you would want.

It is notable that there is so little guidance available for such an important, difficult, and unfamiliar task.

If you can get your doctor to validate your wishes in a letter (confirming that you have discussed this together, and that the doctor considers your wishes to be 'reasonable', especially in the context of any disease you may have), this provides the most powerful sort of planning possible.

This sort of letter provides the profound reassurance that doctors and family really need when they are considering whether they can confidently follow a plan to hold back. Few doctors recognise the value of these letters, so it is important that patients request one.

The doctor writing the letter could be your GP or might be a specialist (you'd know who 'your' doctor is). A doctor's letter also provides confidence that you are not expressing wishes because you are depressed or are being coerced.

These letters are sometimes called treatment plans. Here is an example (the names and situations are fictional):

To whom it may concern,

I am writing this letter to document a discussion that I have had today with Audrey and her daughter Joan.

We talked about Audrey's deteriorating lung function, which is now very limiting. She is unable to do much around the house and she is breathless at the least exertion. The oxygen has not helped much.

Given the precarious situation, we discussed what to do

in a crisis, which I fear is probably just around the corner.

Audrey is clear that she does not want to be 'saved' to continue to deteriorate, but she is very concerned about being frightened and unable to breathe. We discussed a plan to aggressively treat any breathlessness with morphine, and she was very much in favour of this idea.

If it is possible she would like to stay in her own home when her lungs fail, but if this is impractical, she is happy to go to the Colac Hospital, where most of her family will be close. She would not want to be transferred out of Colac.

Joan participated in today's conversation and was understanding of her mother's medical situation and her wishes.

I think this is a very reasonable plan given Audrey's advanced and relentlessly progressive lung disease. She has given it a good go, and I am impressed that she has managed for so long and has kept so cheerful.

I hope that Audrey's lungs hold out for a bit longer, but would be pleased if you are able to implement this plan when the time comes.

With all best wishes,

Dr John Helms, Respiratory Physician

There is often suggestion we simply need tougher legislation to sort everything out: to come up with a 'legal' directive for people to fill out that everyone would have to follow.

Unfortunately, people seem very unwilling to communicate their wishes in this way. Victoria has had a legal 'Refusal of Treatment' form since 1988 that has exactly this legal effect — a doctor can actually be charged with assault if they treat a patient against an instruction on a 'Refusal of Treatment' form.

These forms have been very rarely used over the last 25 years, though. I think I must have seen fewer than five of these forms among the many thousands of patients who have come into intensive care over this time.

Few people feel strongly enough to be willing to formally refuse treatment in this way (despite the fact that most of us recognise that we do have limits). A legalistic approach doesn't seem to match how people actually want to express their wishes, fears, and limits. People seem to want to be *listened* to, and would like their wishes to be recognised and considered. Few choose to do this in a dictating, legal fashion — locking everything up legally seems too inflexible, too strident.

Eva's story

Eva was a grandmother. Her leathery skin was a clear indication of years of wind, sun, and hard work on the family dairy farm.

I first met Eva after she had suffered a respiratory arrest. The arrest hadn't come out of the blue. She had developed a nasty lung disease that had caused relentless scarring of her lungs. As is often the way with these conditions, no treatment over the years seemed to have slowed the progression.

Eva's breathlessness was a major problem. As her lungs had become increasingly scarred, she had been able to do less and less, until the most minimal effort caused her terrible breathlessness. Eva needed continuous oxygen.

I was told that Eva had been determined to stay in her home and had struggled to do so with the help of her husband, Brian.

When Eva arrived in the ICU, she was on a mechanical ventilator. The ambulance crew had arrived at her home just as she stopped breathing. They had expertly passed a breathing tube into her airway, started mechanical ventilation, and rushed her to hospital. There didn't seem to have been any discussion about this course of action, and later enquiry revealed there were no plans in place about what to do in the event of a crisis.

It took a week of intravenous antibiotics to control the pneumonia that had been the last straw for Eva's lungs, but, rather miraculously, we were able to get Eva off the ventilator. She slowly improved to the stage where she started to plan going back home.

I went to see Eva on the ward just before she left hospital. I needed to find out her wishes for when the next crisis hit. For Eva, it wasn't a case of 'if' but 'when' — her lungs were so bad, she was living right on the edge.

It quickly became clear that this was something

that none of her medical team had ever raised with her — certainly not her respiratory specialist (whom she saw regularly), or her GP (whom she saw even more). However, it was also quickly obvious that this was something that Eva worried about a lot. She was scared. Very scared about not being able to breathe, about how she would die. She wasn't scared of being dead — she clearly knew that this was not far away — but she was scared about the bit before that, and worried about what her end would be like.

Eva was very willing to talk to me. She described it as a relief. As far as possible, she wanted to ensure that her end was as easy as it could be. I asked if she would want us to do the same thing next time that had saved her on this occasion — she didn't. She was grateful for our efforts, but reflected that she felt we had 'set her up to go through it all again'. What she wanted was clear — 'to get out without it being too awful'.

I asked her how she would feel about a plan to ensure that the next time her breathing became distressing, we would give her whatever medication might be required to prevent her being uncomfortable or frightened. I was careful to tell her that this treatment might result in her dying, but comfortably. Eva said that it seemed like a great plan, but she was not confident that it could, or would, happen. She surprised me with her insight. She was right to be concerned. It is impossible to promise what others may do. Many doctors and nurses have great reluctance to give medication (however effective at relieving symptoms) that could shorten life.

I wrote of Eva's fears and wishes in her hospital notes. I told her the plan was written down. I urgently organised our advance care planning facilitator to talk to Eva, so that they could formally document her wishes and legally appoint Brian as her agent (to help ensure her wishes were followed).

Eva still wasn't convinced that her wish would be followed. She challenged me to do more.

I phoned Eva's GP to try to add his authority to Eva's wishes. He readily admitted that he had been very worried that Eva was close to dying, but said that he had not raised this with her because he 'didn't want to upset her'. (He is far from being the only doctor to think this!)

I told him about Eva's fears and her desire for a rock-solid plan for 'next time'. I asked him if he could write a letter that would incorporate her wishes into a medical plan.

He agreed that a plan to ensure comfort seemed very reasonable (he said it would be what he'd want if he were in Eva's situation). I asked if he could send me a copy.

He agreed to see Eva as soon as she arrived home that afternoon. He was good to his word. I got an e-mailed copy the next morning.

I had advised Eva that she should distribute the letter widely, so that everyone would be aware of the plan. I also suggested she put a copy in her medicine pack — because ambulance crew always review the drugs someone is on in an emergency and they would find the letter there.

Predictably, Eva did everything I suggested (she was organised and determined).

I later heard that she had lived for four months after she got home. She managed much the same as before her last hospital admission. One evening, she suddenly developed severe breathing difficulty. Brian was with her. He called the GP, but got the answering machine so called the ambulance. They arrived quickly, attended to Eva, found the letter, and confirmed its validity with Brian.

Reassured by the message in the letter, they inserted an intravenous catheter and gave medication to relieve Eva's distress. It worked well. She quickly settled and peacefully passed away.

Some weeks later, Brian came to see me. It's good when relatives feel able to come back and reflect, and I was grateful that he came. He told me that Eva's last months had been that much better because she felt confident that she 'had a clear plan' for the 'bad bit at the end'.

Eva's worry that her original plan would not be enough was fully justified.

Let's think through what could be in doubt when a doctor (or a family member) looks at a plan:

What does this person's doctor think — do they agree or do they violently disagree with the plan? Is any disagreement on the basis that they don't believe the patient was competent to make the plan, or that they had adequate understanding of their medical situation?

What do this person's family think — do they all agree or do some disagree with the plan? Is any disagreement because they believe the patient may have been coerced when they made the plan, or do they doubt their relative's competency to make the plan?

These are common and legitimate concerns that stop plans being confidently followed. No doctor, paramedic, or family member would ever want to let someone die only to find out they incorrectly interpreted a plan or wishes.

It helps to have confidence that everyone is 'on board'. Agreement between the doctor, the patient, and (all) the family that the plan is the 'right' thing is reassuring. It is so reassuring to hear a family say, 'we are all agreed that Mum would never want this', and unsettling to hear that, 'we think that Mum would never want this, but our brother thinks she deserves a chance'.

Theoretically, for someone like Eva who has appointed a substitute decision-maker, it is really only necessary to have the substitute's agreement — but in practice, many doctors (and paramedics) will lack the confidence to hold back life-saving treatment when there are conflicting views.

Because of all these doubts in those who must interpret the wishes in plans, it is wise to go beyond simply creating a plan (or a statement of values and wishes), and to provide more authority to ensure that wishes are followed.

There are several things that can help.

The first is to actively get all the family on side. Ensuring that they know the content of the plan is a good first step; giving them the opportunity to question it is important, too. Their first reaction is often negative. Relatives will not have been thinking about the issues, and it often comes as a surprise. It may simply require reassurance that you have deeply thought about the issues and this is really what you want. Where more is required, you may consider appealing to love — *if you love me, please respect that this is what I want. It is really important to me that you do this for me …*

Many of us try to avoid conflict, so when we know that something is going to cause conflict, we avoid bringing it up. Consequently, plans don't get discussed with 'difficult' relatives. As a result, these relatives are never locked into the plan. But difficult relatives don't go away, and are generally more than willing to express their view (loudly and firmly) when a crisis arises. Dissenting relatives can easily wreck any possibility of a confident decision 'to let go'. There really needs to be effort to get these relatives to respect your right to choose, even if they can't agree with your choice. It may be prudent to specifically exclude this relative from the decision-making process — it is just as valid to exclude someone as it is to select them as decision-maker. I would advise including some positive stuff in the message to minimise any hurt that may be caused. Aggressive, unreasonable people are often surprisingly sensitive. Something like 'I admire my son Adrian's financial abilities, but I would prefer that he *not* be involved in my end-of-life decision-making' might be appropriate.

CHAPTER 5

Important influences on end-of-life decision-making

In this section, we will explore how religious and legal influences, the media, and the human propensity to gamble can affect end-of-life decision-making.

Death is such an important and central aspect of life that it gets a lot of consideration in various religions.

Religions have a lot to say about what we should and shouldn't do, particularly when it comes to dying. The views of religious leaders on ethical matters are often widely reported and these views often have influence way beyond their own congregation.

Sanctity of life is a central premise in many religions, and it is often thought that there is a moral (or eternal) benefit when suffering is endured with fortitude.

Most religions have a view about what is 'right', and

advocate in favour of life and of saving life. Death should not be permitted to occur 'before its time', but generally should not, and need not, be artificially prolonged by medical means. The distinction between the prolongation of life (which is morally required) and the prolongation of death (which is not required) is generally unclear;

In 1995, Pope John Paul II wrote in his *Evangelium Vitae*:

> *To forego extraordinary or disproportionate means*
> *[meaning medical intervention] is not the equivalent*
> *of suicide or euthanasia; it rather expresses acceptance*
> *of the human condition in the face of death.*

This suggests that 'extraordinary or disproportionate' treatment (which might be what we have earlier termed as complex, distressing, excessively burdensome, ineffective, 'heroic' treatment) may be refused — but this leaves a moral requirement *not* to refuse 'ordinary' treatments.

And in turn, this creates the difficulty of deciding what constitutes ordinary (proportionate) treatment and what we would consider to be an extraordinary (disproportionate) treatment. There seems to be no clear religious guidance, which means that individual patients, family, doctors, and religious advisors have to decide this for themselves.

Orthodox Jewish teaching generally takes a stronger position on the sanctity of life:

Ariel's story

In 2006, the then Israeli prime minister, Ariel Sharon, suffered a massive stroke, six weeks before his 78th birthday.

It was clear from the start that this was a catastrophic bleed, and senior doctors at the Jerusalem Hadassah Medical Center advised that he should be allowed to die. However, Sharon's sons (Gilad and Omri) insisted that their father be kept alive.

Surgeons operated for seven hours. Following surgery, he never emerged from his coma and was unable to breathe for himself. From that time on, he required mechanical ventilation to keep him alive.

Judaism is a religion governed by law, ancient laws ('halacha') that go back 3500 years. The traditional, observant Jew incorporates these laws into everyday life. These laws cover choices about medical treatment, and they specifically forbid any action that causes death. Discontinuation of an active treatment that is maintaining life (such as mechanical ventilation) is not permitted. This religious law is mirrored in the Israeli legal system, making it illegal (within the Israeli judicial system) to discontinue mechanical ventilation.

As a result, whatever anyone's wishes might have been after the surgery (including any wishes that Ariel may have expressed), this religious-based law mandated that the mechanical ventilation had to continue. He was moved to the Sheba Medical Center, a long-term health-care facility near Tel Aviv, where he remained unconscious and mechanically ventilated, without any obvious improvement, for the next eight years.

In the end, he developed kidney failure.

From the standpoint of a religious law, the moral situation regarding the kidney failure was different from that which applied to the ongoing mechanical ventilation. As a new life-threatening condition, it was permissible never to start life-saving dialysis (not starting a life-saving treatment is permitted under Jewish law) or, once started, it could be stopped. This is because dialysis is an intermittent treatment, necessitating a new decision to 'do it' before each dialysis treatment. This permits a decision 'not to start it' on each new treatment.

On the other hand, mechanical ventilation is deemed to be a continuous treatment so it can only be taken away — something that is not permitted.

It is unclear if dialysis was withheld or withdrawn, but Ariel Sharon died as a result of kidney failure on 11 January 2014.

His son Gilad is reported to have said, 'He's gone; he went when he decided to go.'

Religious interpretations were important determinants of the treatment decision-making. Despite his son's assertion that his father 'decided' when to go, it might be concluded that he had no say at all, while religion dictated rather a lot.

Jewish teaching considers human life to be of infinite value. Because every life has infinite value, no human life can be considered any less valuable than all others, or any part of a life less valuable than another part. This leaves no possibility for discussion based on quality of life.

In common with other religions, Jewish law forbids doing anything that might shorten life — but may take it more literally than is the case for other religions. Any action that could hasten death is prohibited (even simple things like moving the person), but where there is something that is 'preventing the soul from departing' then this impediment to dying can be removed or ceased.

In Israel, stopping mechanical ventilation is illegal on the basis that its removal causes death (religious law influences civil law in Israel). This means that there are many unconscious patients, who will never awaken, on mechanical ventilators for years in Israel, and their families have no right to stop it (and nor does a patient in any advance directive).

A solution has been suggested that involves the addition of a timer to the mechanical ventilator. The timer makes delivering mechanical ventilation more like dialysis. It forces a new decision to continue mechanical ventilation each time the timer runs out, thus requiring action to reset the timer, otherwise the ventilator would stop. An active decision to withdraw an ongoing treatment (illegal and religiously unsanctioned) may be considered to have changed into a decision *not* to reintroduce a treatment that has ceased (legal).

There is an important catch: the timer has to be included when the mechanical ventilation is first started — it is not permitted to add the timer after mechanical ventilation is in progress. Furthermore, not all Jewish religious authorities accept this 'fix'.

In general, major religions see a spiritual value in suffering and associated fortitude. Muslims may have a greater faith than others that God will reward those who patiently suffer without complaint. Catholics are more likely to see virtue in suffering than is the case for Protestants. People with strong religious conviction are more likely to endure suffering and to ascribe value to the experience.

Some Hindus view death as the transition to another life through reincarnation, life in heaven with God, and ultimately, absorption into Brahma (ultimate reality). A 'good' death is considered very important in this process, and a 'bad' death is greatly feared. Concepts of a bad death include aspects that are also considered undesirable in other cultures: extended prolongation of the process, the use of futile, highly technological treatments, and the absence of family.

At the end of life, some devout Hindus detach themselves from material and emotional concerns to prepare for death through prayer and meditation. These individuals may reject pain-relieving medication, fearing it will interfere with their ability to pray. They may also perceive endurance of pain to be a positive thing, enhancing progress towards Brahma.

To a greater or lesser extent, all religions share a belief that 'God will decide', and should be left to decide, when we are to die. A fundamental interpretation of this belief suggests that man has no authority in this decision. This concept is difficult to reconcile with modern medical practice, where every day, decisions are made to use or to forgo life-prolonging treatment. The idea that 'God' is making the decision can seem confusing. There may be debate about the rightness or otherwise of decisions, the morality of doing or not doing, but the timing of death no longer seems fixed. It is clearly something that we can and do influence.

Prolonging death beyond the time that it would naturally have happened (if we did nothing to stop it) is now common.

Most religions accept that treatment is not mandated when it is futile, but take a different position when a treatment is very burdensome, but not entirely without any possibility of effect. Most teach that there is a moral imperative that treatment and illness should be endured.

Where the burden of treatment is excessive (in the opinion of the patient), most religions suggest that there is no absolute obligation to undergo treatment. It comes down to a debate about the exact degree of burden where it becomes acceptable for a person to decline treatment.

Another question concerns whether it is only appropriate to consider the burden of the treatment, or whether the burden of subsequent disabled living or progressive decline may also be a consideration. For example, many frail patients who are maintained on dialysis for end-stage kidney disease eventually conclude that they are no longer deriving adequate benefit from the dialysis treatment (the burden has become greater than the benefit). When they reach this point, many decide to stop dialysis (precipitating death with a few days). In this case, the treatment itself (dialysis) might not be considered by religious authority to be unduly burdensome and, if continued, it would prolong life.

Another example of a decision to reject potentially 'effective' treatment would be a decision to decline neurosurgery. In itself, this sort of surgery would rarely be considered burdensome (the person would be asleep, and the operation might be technically straightforward). However, the outcome might be a certain survival, but with serious disability and extreme dependency.

Once again, the decision would not be based on the burden of treatment but would hinge on the perceived burden of survival. Burden of survival is generally fraught for religious teachings. The religious position that all human life has infinite value (and suffering with fortitude may be virtuous) makes quality judgments impossible.

Recently, I attended a fabulous academic debate between Peter Singer and Charles Camosy in Brisbane. This vividly displayed how differently secular and religious attitudes deal with the dilemma of dying. I'll share my recollection of this with you.

Peter is widely considered to be a leading social philosopher. He is currently the Ira W. DeCamp professor of bioethics at Princeton University, and is laureate professor at the Centre for Applied Philosophy and Public Ethics at the University of Melbourne. Charles is assistant professor of Christian ethics, at Fordham University in the USA. He is a well-regarded and highly influential Catholic academic.

This was a fantastic opportunity to listen to two very articulate protagonists explain and defend two very different positions. Refreshingly, both were highly respectful, focusing on the issues rather than denigrating the other.

The topic they debated was 'the right to die'. Inevitably, the main focus was voluntary euthanasia, but the right to refuse life-saving treatment was also considered.

Peter spoke first. He took a personal perspective, envisioning a time where his quality of life would make his life so unfulfilling that he would want to be permitted to die. He particularly wanted to avoid becoming a burden on his family. He appealed for his personal autonomy to be respected, his right to make his own choices. Who, he asked, could have the right to overrule his wishes? Surely nobody could have more right than him to decide about his life.

Charles spoke next. He talked softly, with quiet compassion. Unsurprisingly, he took a very different view. He spoke of love.

He suggested that Peter's concern for quality of life caused him to miss the reality and the value of the underlying life. He feared that to focus on *quality* of life risked devaluing life (because it values only life that is considered to have quality). He felt this could lead us to devalue everyone whose quality of life is not considered to be perfect.

He agreed that someone might want to die because they feel that life is awful, but suggested that awfulness is a constructed thing. We so easily contribute to the misery of others by neglect and indifference. We have it within our power to alleviate suffering, but we so often fall short.

He observed that if we are loved, valued, and cherished, nothing should be so bad that we can't face it. He contended that love made planning (or wanting) to die illogical and redundant. He went further, saying that nobody should fear becoming a burden because no loving family or caring society would consider those who are sick or disabled to be a burden. He made it clear that (in his view) burden is in the eye of the 'uncaring carer'. It is simply evidence of our failure to care.

Peter responded that he felt very much loved, and had no doubt about how much everyone cared, particularly his family. It was exactly this understanding that made him fear that he might be kept alive much longer than he would want, in situations that he would not want. He worried that they cared so much, they wouldn't be able to let him go. He realised they would find it difficult to hold back without clear permission or instruction from him (which he had given). He wanted them to be permitted to follow his wishes. He acknowledged the positive power of love, but suggested that there were legitimate concerns about the end of life that love could not deal with, things that he worried about.

Charles suggested that Peter's focus on his individual

rights and wishes was selfish. He questioned the notion that to be 'worthwhile', life needed to be pleasurable and productive; on the contrary, he suggested that difficult lives could have the greatest significance. He suggested that the 'new' emphasis on good lives or 'quality' of life reflected the superficiality of modern secular life.

He expressed concern that permitting people to choose to die would result in coercive pressure on the will of others to fight to live 'because they are being told that they aren't valuable'.

After the debate, I reflected at some length on this exchange. It seemed to me that Peter spoke to us as individuals, acknowledging a common concern about deterioration and death. He gave voice to our worry that medical treatment could prolong our dying. He voiced our desire not to reach a point where the downside of life outweighs the good. He also voiced our wish never to become a burden to others, particularly to those we love.

On the other hand, it felt like Charles was speaking to us as 'family'. He tapped into a deep concern that we simply don't care enough; he touched on how every one of us could do so much more to make the lives of those we love so much better. He eloquently explained our reluctance to let anyone go while there remains any possibility that we could make things 'better'. He shone a light on a potent inner angst ... how we could surely do so much more.

The debaters brilliantly revealed how differently the issues appear when we express our own wishes, and when we are required to implement someone else's wishes that we accept their death and stand back.

Charles came across as totally convinced and caring. His appeal to love was clearly genuine, and he was frank about how his Catholic faith underpinned his analysis. It seemed a clear demonstration of how strongly religion influences the way we feel about the decline and dying of others.

Many, who are not religious, resent the degree to which religion dictates choices for others who do not share similar beliefs. From a practical perspective, the important thing is to be able to recognise how religious teaching may be influencing our decisions and those of others (and to be able to accept, reject, or modify the concepts that inform these influences).

The law is also intimately involved in death (mostly in preventing it).

The entire coronial court system is specifically created to identify preventable deaths. The law regards the preservation of life as a fundamental principle. The sanctity of life and protecting the lives of the vulnerable are important legal principles.

Where someone dies, because of something done by someone else, even one minute before they were 'destined' to die, then this is technically murder (whether or not death is the intention of the action or inaction).

Causing death is considered to be among the most serious of crimes. Causing, or failing to prevent, death can easily be construed to be an illegal act.

There are two important legal exceptions: when a competent patient refuses the treatment; and where the treatment is futile or not in the patient's best interest.

Since a charge of murder or manslaughter is very serious, it is important to be clear which of these exceptions is being invoked whenever we decide to stop or withhold (i.e., not to start) any sort of life support.

The first exception (a competent patient refuses treatment or a properly appointed agent has refused on the patient's behalf) is generally self-explanatory. The fact that treatment is unwanted just needs to be clear to everyone and needs to be properly documented.

When the patient is unconscious and has not appointed an agent, the last two criteria (the treatment is futile or the treatment is not in the patient's best interests) are all that are available to guide the decision-making. Unfortunately, both 'futility' and 'best interests' are open to interpretation.

Futility is a difficult concept. The dictionary definition of futility is 'incapable of producing any useful result'. But people can have very different opinions about what is 'useful'.

Let's consider a hypothetical case — a patient with advanced lung cancer who is near to the end and has now developed a severe pneumonia causing dangerously low oxygen levels. Taking over the breathing with mechanical ventilation would almost certainly result in improved circulating oxygen levels — this is a positive physiological effect that might be considered to be useful.

Immediate death would also be prevented — and this might also be considered to be useful.

But with end-stage cancer, this person would almost certainly not ever be able to get off the ventilator, and their death would probably simply be prolonged by the intervention. Looked at this way, there would be no useful long-term benefit.

It's possible to have this sort of debate about whether a treatment is 'futile' in almost every situation. It can often be simpler (and more effective) to focus consideration on what would be, and would not be, in the patient's best interests.

What is in an individual's best interest is most reliably based on what the patient would want. From a legal standpoint, nobody is likely to fall foul of the law when they are considered to be trying to act in the best interests of the patient.

There is a clear legal approach to establishing what an unconscious (or otherwise incompetent) person might want — this provides a robust process for family and doctors to follow, even when the court is not involved.

First, there is a need to find out both the *fact* of the person's wishes (what they have said) together with consideration of the *circumstances* that surrounded the expression of these wishes (how the person was thinking when they expressed them).

In general, written evidence is afforded more weight than oral evidence, because lawyers believe that the formality associated with writing, signing, and getting a document witnessed indicates a greater intent than is the case for an informal oral statement.

A second consideration is how old the statement is. Where it is very old, it is reasonable to question whether the expressed wishes accurately represent the person's current wishes.

Third, the formal appointment of a substitute decision-maker is seen to carry significant legal weight, since this is an indication that the patient 'wants' this person to make treatment decisions for them, and has used a formal legal process to express trust in them and their decisions.

When trying to determine the validity of a patient's wishes, lawyers consider how certain they need to be about the person's wishes (this is termed 'standard of proof' in legal terminology).

The standard of proof would be higher if the statement was applicable to the current context, seemed to be considered, was unambiguous and repeated, was consistent with a pattern of similar decisions, and was in character. This seems a very reasonable way to assess the validity of statements.

For example, imagine trying to establish the wishes of a woman who has been in an accident and is now in a persistent coma. A family member reports that her mother, the patient, had said, 'Were I ever unable to communicate, and there was little chance of improvement, I wouldn't want to be kept alive.' This would be quite specific to the current circumstances and seems considered. Where such an opinion was consistent with the mum's character, it would be reasonable to give some weight to this statement.

A lawyer would also want to be assured that the family member reporting the mum's wish was not acting with an ulterior motive, such as wishing to avoid having to care for their incapacitated mum, or the desire to access an inheritance.

Having established the patient's wishes, to the best of his or her ability, a lawyer would then consider whether there was an adequate degree of certainty concerning these wishes.

Courts generally believe that the degree of certainty needs to be higher in situations where the significance of the decision to be made is very important. Since not providing life-saving treatment usually results in death, this decision is considered to be very important. As a result, the legal approach demands that no decision should be made (to withhold treatment) without a high degree of certainty that this is *really* what the person would want.

From a legal perspective, a balance of probability, or a consensus by the family of what is the best interest of the patient, would represent an inadequate basis for such an important decision.

While this is important to recognise, it is also important to realise that it is almost impossible to achieve the degree of certainty that a court would require — and very few cases go to court (especially where there is consensus between the family and doctors).

In regard to the degree of certainty that is commonly

available, consider the following rather typical, and common, scenario.

Susan's story

Susan was a 79-year-old widow. She had retired to a beachside suburb, and was in hospital after suffering a major stroke.

The stroke was a catastrophe that had followed a long period of slow progressive physical and mental deterioration (most probably related to a series of small strokes).

Susan's eyes sometimes seemed to track the movement of people in the room, and she grimaced when turned in bed. She had a poor cough reflex and was unable to cough sputum from her chest. The ambulance crew had inserted a breathing tube when they found her collapsed at home, so, in hospital, the sputum was being suctioned through this tube.

Susan was able to maintain her breathing, so the mechanical support was progressively weaned off.

An experienced neurologist told Susan's adult children that Susan had no realistic prospect of significant improvement; what she actually said was 'as close to no chance as I can come'.

She explained that there was a choice to make.

If a tracheostomy tube was inserted into Susan's neck, then the sputum could continue to be effectively suctioned. If this were done, then Susan would probably survive to go to a high-level nursing home (where she might live for some time).

If the breathing tube were to be removed, then Susan would be unable to cough the sputum out. Pneumonia would quickly develop (probably within days), and this would likely kill her. Medication could be given to avoid discomfort.

The children were asked what they thought that their mother would want.

They all agreed that their mother was always an interested, interactive, and active woman. They thought that she would find it intolerable to be so dependent.

They also shared that they 'hate seeing her like this'.

They requested the tube be removed, that no tracheostomy be performed, and that she be kept comfortable.

A legal expectation that there be a high standard of certainty regarding Susan's wishes would mean that the general comments the family offered about Susan (things about her, rather than specific wishes applicable to this particular situation) would fail this requirement. The children also expressed their feelings (they 'hate seeing her like this') rather than presenting their mother's interest and wishes. Personal opinions of family members tell us nothing directly about Susan's wishes. Furthermore, courts are generally suspicious of the needs and wants of 'others' when coming to decisions about medical treatments.

So a legal opinion might well conclude that this family should not be empowered to make a decision to palliate (or 'not to save', as they might construe it). A lawyer might consider that this decision should be referred to a statutory authority to decide (such as a tribunal or a court). In reality, these sorts of decisions are made many times every day in hospitals, nursing homes, and in patients' homes across the country. These decisions often have to be made rapidly. Despite the obvious difficulty, and inherent ambiguity, the vast majority of decisions are loving, considered, collaborative, appropriate, reasonable, and uncontested. It is unlikely that any court could do a better job — and most lawyers know this.

Very substantial resources would be required if legal involvement was mandated in each and every case. Courts are remote from the patient and the family. Lawyers and court officials are generally unable to visit (due to time and resource limitations), and when they *do* visit patients, they encounter the same problem as everyone else — they are unable to communicate with the person, and uncertain how much to trust what the family are saying.

On top of this, legal processes are protracted (in part, due to the time needed to collect and evaluate all possible relevant information), delayed (due to the restraints on court time), and expensive. Requiring a legal process is liable to lead to prolongation of a situation that may already be considered to be unacceptably distressing and degrading.

Inevitably, those cases that *do* end up going to court get the advantage of very detailed and extensive consideration. The resulting judgments are important, as they can provide useful guidance to inform decisions for the many cases that do not end up in court. For this reason, we might usefully look at some recent rulings in some detail:

The Messiha case

On 17 October 2004, 75-year-old Isaac Messiha was admitted to the intensive care unit (ICU) of St George Hospital in New South Wales.

He had suffered an out-of-hospital cardiac arrest. Resuscitation attempts had been started only when the ambulance officers arrived. It was estimated that his brain had been deprived of oxygen for over 25 minutes after his heart stopped (an awfully long time).

From the start, the ICU staff and neurology specialists were worried that such a prolonged period without blood flow to the brain would have caused severe damage.

Isaac had no formal advance directive and had not formally appointed anyone to make medical decisions for him.

Over the next few days, he did not waken or improve (consistent with the doctors' assessment of the severity of his brain injury).

The family was informed of the medical opinion that

there was no realistic prospect of a return to a meaningful quality of life. Subsequent electroencephalography (EEG) showed the absence of cortical activity (confirming that the brain damage was very severe indeed).

At this time, Isaac was being mechanically ventilated, was being fed through a tube into his stomach, had a catheter to drain his urine, was incontinent of faeces, and required regular suctioning of saliva and sputum.

The doctors proposed that it would be in Isaac's best interests that further treatment be withheld, and that the treatment he was getting should be discontinued.

Isaac's relatives strongly disagreed and arranged for an independent neurologist to give a second opinion. This opinion supported the view of the local doctors.

The relatives then sought an order from the Supreme Court of New South Wales to prevent the medical treatment from being withdrawn.

The court respected the medical assessment and decided that the decision to discontinue treatment was in Isaac's best interest — despite the family's contrary opinion.

The life support treatment was discontinued and Isaac died soon after.

The Schiavo case

On 25 February 1990, Terri Schiavo suffered severe brain damage after suffering a prolonged cardiac arrest.

Low potassium levels in the blood — caused by the anorexia from which Terri suffered — were thought to have caused the arrest.

This happened in the USA (which may help explain some of the later events).

After some months, with no improvement in her conscious state, her neurologists diagnosed Terri to be in an irreversible Persistent Vegetative State. She remained unchanged over a number of subsequent years.

Eventually, her husband, Michael (her legal guardian), applied to the court to be permitted to request discontinuation of his wife's tube feeding. Terri's parents, who were devout Catholics, opposed this.

This led to ongoing legal wrangling with more than 25 court cases over the next 10 years. Catholic organisations, including the Vatican, supported Terri's parents' position. It all ended up with an extraordinary sitting of the US Congress, who referred the case to the federal court.

Finally, the highest court ruled against the parents' application and, late in March 2005, the feeding tube was removed, and Terri died (15 years after her cardiac arrest).

It is worth noting that in the USA, there is a far greater emphasis on 'substituted' judgment than is the case in many other countries. This means that *what the person is thought to have wanted* is considered to be much more important than what may be considered to be in their best interests. In the USA, a substitute decision-maker needs to provide 'clear and convincing' evidence of what the patient would want — which is challenging when they have said nothing about what they might want in a particular situation (as in Terri's case).

The Thompson case

John Thompson was a 37-year-old man who suffered a cardiac arrest, thought to have been due to a heroin overdose. He was taken to the Royal Prince Alfred Hospital in Sydney after being resuscitated at the roadside.

He remained unconscious.

His situation remained unchanged six days later. John displayed neurological signs that led the medical staff to conclude that any neurological recovery would be very poor. They concluded that it would be in John's best interest to cease artificial feeding and antibiotic treatment. The medical team presented this plan to John's mother. It is reported that she seemed shocked but said little. She contacted her daughter, John's sister ('Mrs Northridge' in the law report), who strongly objected to the plan.

The family felt that John could survive if he were provided with 'proper' medical care. John's sister contacted the medical team to ask for her brother's medical treatment to be resumed and to oppose a 'Not

For Resuscitation' order that had been placed on her brother. After she failed to convince the medical staff, she appealed to the Supreme Court of NSW, who subsequently intervened.

During the ensuing court proceedings, it became evident that John's neurological condition had improved since the initial assessment.

The court ruled that John should be provided with 'all necessary and appropriate' medical treatment for the 'preservation of his life and the promotion of his good health and welfare' as long as he remained in hospital. It was also ordered that no 'Not-For-Resuscitation' order was to be made without the court's authority.

The hospital followed the orders of the court.

John survived. However, his neurological injury proved to be very significant. He remained totally dependent for all care, and he was discharged to high-level nursing-home care. He has remained there ever since.

The Bland case

Tony Bland was a young football supporter who was tragically injured in the 1989 Hillsborough disaster in the UK (where Liverpool Football Club supporters were crushed by overcrowding, resulting in the deaths of 96 people).

During the crush, Tony was deprived of oxygen for a long period, which caused irreparable brain injury and left him in a Persistent Vegetative State. Every doctor who examined Tony agreed with this assessment, and none felt that that there was any prospect of improvement.

Tony's family was very attentive and visited him regularly. But after years of seeing no change in his condition, they came to question the value of continued medical support.

Following discussion between the family and the staff caring for Tony, there was unanimous agreement that treatment, including tube feeding, was no longer in Tony's best interest and should be discontinued.

Since there were ongoing investigations into the disaster, with significant media interest, the senior doctor managing the case (Dr Howe) informed the coroner of the decision before discontinuing the artificial feeding. The coroner made it clear that he '... could not countenance, condone, approve or give consent to any action or inaction which could be, or could be construed as being, designed or intended to shorten or terminate the life of this young man. This particularly applies to the withholding of the necessities of life, such as food and drink'.

As well as sending this message, the coroner requested a reply (by return) notifying him that Dr Howe had understood his opinion, and would not withdraw treatment. The coroner also sent copies of his letter to the police, the solicitor for the Regional Health Authority, and to Dr Howe's medical defence organisation (insurer).

The following day, Dr Howe was visited by a detective from the local Criminal Investigation Department (CID) who informed him that, were he to withdraw treatment and Tony died, then he would be charged with murder!

In light of the coroner's response, the Health Authority made plans to apply to the court for permission to lawfully terminate medical treatment.

At this stage, Tony's family felt that they could not face court proceedings (the media attention up to that time had been intense) so they did not consent to the application being made. All support continued, although the family were upset about this and felt that it was 'not right'.

Eventually, the family did consent to an application being made to the court and after extensive legal consideration (which eventually reached the House of Lords), it was concluded that support could be discontinued. This ruling was upheld on appeal.

Tube feeding was discontinued, and Tony died.

The BWV case

(The patient's name was suppressed in the legal case and she was only ever referred to as BWV, so we will use this abbreviation in our review of the case.)

BWV was a 68-year-old Melbourne woman who had an unusual form of progressive dementia known as Pick's disease.

Eight years earlier, when she was already unable to communicate, make decisions, or swallow, a PEG tube had been inserted so she could be fed directly into her stomach.

During the three years before the case came to court, BWV was bedridden, lying in a contracted position, and able to move nothing but her eyes. She did not appear to be conscious of anything in her environment and did not interact in a meaningful way.

The medical opinion was unanimous that there was no prospect of recovery or improvement, and also that her current condition was not a situation that she would have wanted. They believed that continued provision of nutrition and hydration was inappropriate and should stop. The family agreed.

BWV had not appointed substitute medical decision-maker, so the Office of the Public Advocate was asked to conduct an investigation of BWV's wishes regarding treatment.

BWV's husband and children reported that she had made it clear to them (when she was still competent) that she would not want medical treatment to keep her alive in the face of such debility. The family requested that feeding be stopped, and at that time, it was not clear, legally, that the hospital could do this (even if they agreed that it would be medically appropriate). There was (and still is) opinion that the provision of food and drink are basic human rights, and that it is wrong to withhold them. On the other hand, others believe there are circumstances where continuation of food and water confer no benefit and can reasonably be stopped.

It was concluded that the feeding itself was unlikely to result in such distress as to justify its discontinuation — so the decision needed to rest on evidence that BWV would not want this treatment.

The public advocate was appointed as guardian. The court decided that the provision of artificial nutrition and hydration 'involves protocols, skills, and care which draw from and depend upon medical knowledge' and concluded that tube feeding was 'a medical procedure'.

As a medical procedure, the court then went on to decide that artificial feeding and nutrition could be lawfully refused, and that the public advocate could make the decision to refuse it if he felt this would be what BWV wanted.

The public advocate made that decision.

Feeding and hydration through the PEG tube were discontinued, and BWV died.

Margaret Tighe who was, at the time, president of the Right to Life (Australia) organisation commented that it was 'not an act of love to kill somebody by dehydration and starvation'.

The Catholic Archbishop of Melbourne observed that it was his belief that the law (as enacted by parliament) had never intended that 'elderly, handicapped, and unconscious people, who were not dying, should be deprived of food and water'.

These cases illustrate the gravity with which withdrawal or withholding of treatment are seen, as well as the detail that the courts apply when reaching a decision to discontinue life support.

Similar legal determinations have now been made in many countries, but the arguments are ongoing. Those who agree with the idea that a feeding tube is a medical intervention are likely to consider its continuation, in irreversibly unconscious patients, to be both undignified and pointless. While those who perceive the tube simply as a logical continuation of the basic act of feeding are likely to view it as a simple act of humanity, something that we are all morally bound to continue.

On the basis of existing legal judgments, it seems that courts will rarely act against unanimous medical opinion that prolonged life support is contrary to the interests of a terminally ill patient in a deep coma, who has no realistic prospect of recovery.

On the other hand, in cases of severe but not 'hopeless' neurological injury, a demand for ongoing medical support by relatives (even where this is contrary to medical opinion) may be upheld. However, family demands are likely to be overruled where there is clear evidence that the patient would not want such treatment.

There are a number of situations where courts have

agreed that permitting death is preferable to ongoing medical support, including the following: where death will be inevitable in the short term, whatever therapy is provided; where there is an unequivocal diagnosis of Persistent Vegetative State or very severe brain damage (where there is no possibility of 'meaningful interactive life'); and where there is interminable pain and suffering with the prospect of a demonstrably awful life.

It is important to remember that legal judgments relate to the specific case that was under consideration, and may not necessarily apply to similar, but different, situations. For instance, where the severity of the medical condition is different, the perceived distress is different, or where the person's expressed wishes are expressed in a different way.

It is also important to note that these standards have often been applied by the courts in the context of conflict between family members or between the family and the hospital. When there is conflict, the level of confidence required for a decision to discontinue support would likely be higher than would be the case when there is a consensus.

The media is another big influence. They love sensational stories of medical miracles. Stories of triumph against impossible odds, preferably against medical advice, are encouraging, inspiring, and uplifting. They can't get enough (and the readership lap them up).

These stories raise expectations. They suggest that we should be hopeful in the face of impossible odds, and that it is right to dismiss advice and fact. The message we see every day in the media supports never accepting, never giving up, and trying against the odds.

Stories of pragmatism are rarely exciting enough to get a mention, so there is little media support for any sort of realistic acceptance.

Depiction of cardiopulmonary resuscitation (CPR) is a good example of media distortion. To look at the message portrayed on television, a group of researchers observed CPR outcomes on popular US medical television programs including *ER*, *Chicago Hope*, and *Rescue 911*.

They observed that 75 per cent of the patients survived the immediate arrest, with 67 per cent appearing to survive intact to hospital discharge.

This contrasts starkly with reality, where only 5–10 per cent survive, and many of them are left with serious neurological injury. Of course, the patients portrayed on the television were also much younger and fitter than in reality.

Media reporting of the Terri Schiavo case (reviewed earlier) also provides a good example of how media can distort or confuse in the interests of sensationalism. In Terri's case, there was undisputed agreement that she was suffering from Persistent Vegetative State (PVS). In PVS, the person never shows evidence of any meaningful response to their surroundings (they can't, because they are completely unaware). Terri's eventual post mortem confirmed she had the sort of massive brain damage that is characteristic of PVS, so there was no justification to have doubted this. The issue under consideration by the courts (that the press were supposed to be reporting) was not to dispute the diagnosis. The issue that the courts were asked to consider was whether Terri would want medical care to maintain her indefinitely in this state or, failing to establish her wishes, whether it would be in her best interest to be maintained in this way.

The media reported it very differently. In the newspaper articles about the case, the implications of PVS (not being aware, never waking up) were rarely discussed, featuring in only about 1 per cent of articles. Over 20 per cent suggested that Terri 'might improve' and 7 per cent suggested that she 'might recover'. Many attributed conscious behaviour to Terri that would be completely implausible in someone with PVS. These included reports that Terri was able to respond (10 per cent of articles), smile (5 per cent of articles), and laugh (5 per cent of articles).

Many articles included emotive language to describe the contemplated withdrawal of feeding. Nearly 10 per cent of articles described discontinuation of artificial nutrition and hydration as 'murder'.

The media coverage added significant confusion and tension, rather than disseminating information that might help readers clarify the issues and make their own judgment on the merits (or otherwise) of the arguments that were before the courts.

This sort of medical misreporting is unfortunate, as the public increasingly depends on the media for education about medicine and ethics. Sadly, in the future, it is likely that sensationalism will only increase.

Beyond traditional media, the actual words we use when we talk about death and disease are important influences on how we behave. The way we express things directs and restricts how we think.

As we speak of fighting, of overcoming, of battling, of beating the odds — we construct a narrative where 'doing' becomes logical and expected, and where 'not doing' is actively excluded.

When we choose to say, 'if you are near death' or 'if you were to get very sick' rather than 'when you are near death' or 'when you were to get very sick', we construct a narrative that suggests that such situations aren't inevitable and can be ignored.

Finding language that describes disease and dying in ways that do not actively promote intervention can be challenging (because the words we use are so charged).

Furthermore, different diseases get talked about, and thought about, very differently. Cancer is generally presented with a battle narrative, while kidney failure is discussed as a chore. People aren't described as 'battling' their kidney failure, or their liver failure. They live with it. Those who survive for a long time with kidney failure generally don't refer to themselves as 'survivors'. However, the treatment for kidney failure may be more arduous than that for cancer, and outcomes are often worse.

No discussion of influences would be complete without also looking at ourselves and considering how gambling influences our choices.

Gambling is clearly a major human failing — we lose so much and yet we keep on doing it. Australians gamble more per capita than any other nation and lost a stunning $23 billion gambling in 2016, a figure that says nothing encouraging about our ability to deal with probability in any rational way.

We react to gains and losses very differently. We like to win, but we really dislike losing. The reaction to loss is called *loss aversion*. Imagine you go to the casino, bet $50, and lose. Would you cut your losses and leave? Probably not. Almost everyone chooses to continue to gamble to try to win back the lost $50. There's a chance you might win it back, but, as the odds are against you, it is more likely you will lose more. With the first bet, you were hoping to win, but with the second bet, motivation has changed to trying to recoup a loss. Because we hate loss, we find it very difficult to give up in the face of previous losses.

It's easy to see how this attitude to loss relates to decisions to escalate treatment efforts when previous treatments have failed. The motivation is so much greater when a lot has been invested (when the failed treatment was very unpleasant).

The lottery is a bit different. Here, we discount the insignificant price of the lottery ticket as we focus on the glittering possibility that we may win. Our brain lets us down again. The chance of winning the lottery is vanishingly unlikely, but we think about winning as though it will definitely happen to us. Here is the power of possibility again.

Having a lottery ticket opens up possibilities — psychologists describe this as having a 'higher ceiling of possibility'. Having the ticket makes things possible (in our imagination) that were impossible before we had the ticket. This effect is greater for those who have limited possibilities, because this high ceiling is that much more attractive to those who had nothing (this explains why the highest gambling losses occur in the poorest suburbs and among those who are in the worst situation). Hoping that treatment will work against the odds has a lot in common with buying a lottery ticket.

Possibility tells us that *someone* has to win — and it could be you. It is easy (and pleasurable) to image how you might feel if you won. The mental image of winning is vivid, attractive, and emotional.

Probability tells us that we are vanishingly unlikely to win, as the odds of winning are so very, very low. However, the feelings associated with losing are much less vivid, much less attractive, and not emotional at all. We don't enjoy thinking about losing, and so it tends to get suppressed or ignored.

As we ignore the thought of losing, the vision of winning easily comes to dominate our thinking. We are not balancing the risk of loss with the chance of winning; we're just dreaming of winning.

This propensity to overrate our chances of winning isn't

that much of a problem when the stakes are low, but it becomes a real problem when there is a lot to lose. This is unfortunately how it is when we gamble with increasingly burdensome treatment in the face of very little chance of success.

Dealing rationally with risk involves confronting the issues with eyes wide open, avoiding the temptation to be unduly influenced by the possibility of success, and giving adequate consideration to probability.

It comes down to balancing optimism with fact, and hope with reality.

How we frame choices also has great influence. The way that information is presented to us has a major influence on what we end up choosing.

In a classic study in 1982, participants were asked to imagine they had lung cancer and were told they had a choice of two therapies: radiation or surgery. They were told either that 32 per cent of patients were dead one year after having radiation, or that 68 per cent of patients were alive one year after having radiation.

These are just different ways of presenting *exactly the same information* (they add up to 100 per cent).

What happened? Well, 44 per cent of those who were given the information about the one-year *survival* chose radiation, compared to only 18 per cent of those who were given the one-year *mortality* figure. Giving the positive (survival) information more than doubled the number selecting the treatment.

This study is important, because it shows just how much

the way medical information is presented affects the choices that we make.

Even more remarkably, the study showed that doctors were just as influenced as everyone else (about a third of the participants in the survey were doctors). It seems that clinical experience and medical knowledge doesn't protect us from the effect of 'positive spin'.

We all need to be on a constant lookout to try to ensure that we are assessing chances and risks reasonably.

CHAPTER 6

Practical tips

The most important tip is to anticipate how doctors think.

At my hospital, we regularly run an interesting experiment with our new trainees. We tell them about a patient on the ward whom the medical team are pushing to have admitted to the ICU. We give them enough detail to make it clear that this (hypothetical) patient has minimal chance of survival (even with full ICU care) and, if they were to survive, that they would have a long, complicated stay in the ICU. We also tell them that, if the patient did manage to pull through, they would be left much worse off than before, requiring high-level nursing-home care.

We tell them that they have to decide whether or not to admit the patient to the ICU …

What we are presenting them with is an increasingly common, very difficult, 'lose-lose' situation. The choice here is between two awful options.

There is no clear 'right' answer. It would not be wrong to admit this patient to the ICU (if the patient really wanted to try), nor would it be wrong keep the patient on the ward, and ensure a comfortable death (if the patient prefers this).

All the doctors recognise that we are presenting them with a difficult problem — but it's one that they will encounter on a daily basis.

We tell them that they have *three* questions to help them to decide which way to go. We want to see how they use their wishes as this provides insight into how they are thinking about the problem.

We have found that there are three main categories of questions they ask:

The first is to ask for more medical information, suggesting that they are thinking about the disease — *What does the chest X-ray show? Is the white-cell count raised?* — that sort of thing.

The second is to ask what others (other than the patient) want or expect: *What does the surgeon expect? What do the family want?*

The third category involves a range of questions about what the patient wants or values — what *they* think is important or unacceptable.

How do you think the doctors use their questions?

Almost all of them use up *all* their questions trying to get more medical information. Some use one or two to find out what others want; usually, they want to know what the family wants.

Few use *any* of their questions to find out what the patient wants!

We go on to discuss why they approach the problem in this way. This leads us to explain how understanding the patient's wishes and priorities is generally the only way to resolve this sort of dilemma. This seems to come as a major revelation to most of them. We train them how to listen, and thus to understand what is important to patients. We hope that, through this, we can prepare them to be much better doctors throughout their careers. It's our legacy.

However, it will take time, and for now you would be well advised to assume that any doctors you meet will focus on medical issues rather than on the patient's wishes, and it will be important to ensure that there is focus on patient wishes by the family bringing this up.

There is a common medical belief that nobody (who is not suicidal) would ever reasonably want to die until every possible treatment option has been completely and utterly exhausted. This makes it seem inappropriate for the doctor to consider any wishes that a patient might have expressed until all treatment has been tried and failed. Comments such as 'We're not at that stage', 'First we have to be sure that the treatment's not working', and 'It's too early to think about that' all suggest this attitude.

It should never be too early to consider what a patient wants; patients' wishes should underpin everything we do. When the doctor doesn't ask, it is important that patients and family ensure that wishes, fears, and values are presented and considered.

Gavin's mum's story

Gavin and I have worked together over many years. Gavin is an excellent, highly experienced nurse. I never met Gavin's mum, but Gavin has told me about her and her medical experiences. It's obviously something that has had a profound effect on him.

(Gavin's mum has a name, but since in our conversations she has always been 'Gavin's mum', it seems appropriate to keep this convention here.)

Like many, Gavin's mum was active and relatively well into her early 80s. Then she got an irritating cough that wouldn't go away. An X-ray showed widespread cancer throughout her lung. This turned out to be an aggressive, inoperable alveolar cell cancer.

This type of cancer can cause massive fluid secretion into the airway, particularly in the later stages of disease. This is what happened to Gavin's mum, and it proved particularly distressing.

As the end approached, this fluid became more and more of a problem. Her strength failed and her cough became weaker, while the amount of secretion increased.

She was drowning.

It all got too much. She asked Gavin to take her to the hospital. The doctor who saw her organised a CT scan, blood tests, an ECG, and an ultrasound of her chest.

It wasn't what she wanted. She got Gavin to take her home. He was distraught; he tried to get her to stay, but she insisted. He did as she asked.

She had a terrible night, and the next day, she went back to hospital. This time, she was seen by a young specialist whom we know well. He had trained with us.

Once he had done a basic assessment, he pulled up a chair, held her hand, and asked what she was most worried about. He recognised the importance of finding out about her fears, goals, and priorities.

She cried. Gavin cried. It all came out.

Knowing what she wanted, the specialist was then able to provide the care she needed.

Saving is what doctors do — this is felt as a very profound commitment.

However, in our training, we wanted our junior doctors to be more honest and to offer choice. We gave them a scenario where escalation was reasonable (to do everything possible to save) and palliation was reasonable (to focus on comfort and to let death occur). We asked the doctors to outline two options (treatment or palliation) and then to use their listening skills to work out which option the patient preferred.

We expected that they would find this task quite straightforward.

We were wrong. Few of them could get past the explanation bit. They presented the treatment option without difficulty (though most made light of the implications of the intense treatment required). But they struggled to offer palliation. They fidgeted, looked at the floor, they looked uneasy, they scrambled their words, they used euphemisms that totally obscured what they were saying. When we asked, the actors had no doubt that the doctor talking to them did not favour palliation and had strongly recommended intervention (to save).

When we asked the doctors why they found it so difficult, they told us that they felt it was wrong to raise the possibility of palliation when there was still a chance that treatment could work.

This was obviously something we needed to talk about. They had just agreed that every patient has the right to forgo treatment that they don't want. Most had also agreed that *they* would probably choose to be palliated in the situation that they were describing. They recognised that it was their duty to provide patients with information about *all* the available options, so they were able make a proper informed decision … but then they found that they couldn't do it.

Despite their theoretical agreement with the concept of giving choice, it seemed that they felt uncomfortable putting the possibility of palliation 'on the table' until attempts to save had clearly failed. One of the doctors summarised their approach when she said, 'If I put it out there the patient might pick it up and they wouldn't get to try treatment.'

It is clearly a potent concern for these doctors.

A similar attitude lay behind a complaint I received from an oncologist. He was upset that our junior doctors were talking to his very sick (dying) patients when they presented to ICU in crisis. Our doctors were raising the possibility of palliation or of setting limits to how far to push treatment.

He felt it was quite inappropriate for the junior staff to mention palliation at all before *he* had reached the stage where he had no more treatment to offer. He expressed concern that 'all' his patients would select comfort in preference to what he was offering! I don't think he has changed his position. He is far from being unique.

There is some fascinating and important psychology that needs to be understood and untwined. This must be an important focus for future research.

For now, it seems that patients and families can assume that their doctor will advocate treatment that has curative intent (even were they to believe this burdensome and unlikely to work). It will be left to patients and families to ensure that the possibility of a focus on comfort is discussed (even though it may not turn out to be the best choice).

While families can assist good decision-making, they can also sabotage it. Again, there are many examples, but Rosalie stands out.

Rosalie's story

Rosalie was an elderly lady who lived on a farm in a remote area. She had been deteriorating for years and had become almost entirely dependent on her only daughter, May, for all her care.

May had never married, and she had given up a well-paid job five years earlier to look after her mother. She had looked after Rosalie amazingly well.

May and her mum were obviously very close. Rosalie's husband, Bob (May's dad), had died ten years earlier. As Rosalie's health failed, she chose May to be her agent (her legally appointed substitute decision-maker).

Rosalie arrived at our hospital with a very serious, deep, overwhelming infection. It involved her groin area and an extensive part of her left leg. It was immediately clear that this would most likely prove unsurvivable (in view of its extent, the severity of symptoms, and Rosalie's poor general health and frailty). In the unlikely event that Rosalie did survive, it would involve massive and repeated surgery, a very prolonged hospital stay, and would result in further deterioration in Rosalie's level of dependency.

All this was discussed with May (Rosalie was much too sick to participate). We came to a very clear decision that the best thing for Rosalie would be not to escalate to burdensome treatment, as it would cause Rosalie significant discomfort without offering meaningful benefit. We agreed to ensure her comfort.

It seemed reasonable. May seemed to be clearly

and sensitively representing her mother's interests. May told us how frustrated Rosalie had become and how concerned she was about becoming worse.

It all seemed straightforward. How wrong you can be!

May's brothers arrived. There were five of them. May was the youngest of six children, and the only girl. The brothers were united. Their mum had to be saved. They felt that May was deluded, weak, and didn't understand.

Shortly afterwards, May asked for a further meeting with the medical team. She told us that she had changed her mind. She wanted 'everything done to save Mum'.

She seemed a different person. She gave no reason for her change of mind, but she seemed frightened. She didn't want to talk about it. She became visibly upset when we asked her how she felt this new decision fitted with what she had told us of Rosalie's wishes and concerns.

We never got any further. May was the decision-maker — and she had changed her mind. That was it. We had concerns that she was misguided and was being unduly influenced by her brothers, but she denied it.

We kept Rosalie on life support for weeks. She went to surgery six times. She got a tracheostomy. Eventually, she developed progressive failure of multiple organs. Much of the time, she had to have her arms restrained to stop her from pulling out all her tubes.

Finally, Rosalie died.

Throughout, May remained withdrawn and uncommunicative. She seemed crushed and guilty.

I often wonder about the long-term effect this experience had on her.

This was a stark and very unfortunate case. I'm sure that Rosalie would have been very distressed if she had known what her sons had done to her (and to May).

Unfortunately, this sort of thing happens rather often. When we exclude family members from decision-making (or don't choose them), they can still exert influence and it can even motivate them to do so! To prevent this it is important to inform everyone (who might assume responsibility) of wishes, and to obtain reassurance that they will respect wishes.

The message is clear — the more dysfunctional and the more unlikely family are to respect wishes, the *more important* it is to get everyone to promise to behave. I've no doubt that Rosalie would agree.

Sometimes families do quite the opposite, providing clear respect for wishes and great support to decision-makers. Solidarity in the family becomes particularly important when the doctor/s are unwilling to listen. Ben's case was like that.

Ben's story

Ben was an elderly farmer. He had had a small stroke some months before. Although the stroke hadn't been too bad, it had a devastating effect on him. He couldn't get into the tractor and couldn't drive. From his perspective, this had been a disaster. Ben's frustration at the time had been very obvious. It clearly mattered to Ben to be able to run his farm and, unable to do so, he was devastated. He didn't read and watched little TV.

After he recovered, surgery was performed to prevent him suffering a more serious stroke. This seemed like a good idea, based on the effect the stroke had had on him, but as soon as he woke up, it was clear that he'd suffered a massive stroke during the surgery. Over the next few days, the extent became clear, and it was bad. The scans were terrible. A neurology consult reported that there was 'no realistic chance of a good recovery' and that it was likely that Ben would require 'long-term high-level nursing-home care' if he were to survive. The family were informed.

The surgeon arranged to meet Ben's wife and daughter (Ben couldn't communicate). The surgeon wanted the family to consent to a tracheostomy and a PEG feeding tube. I sat in on the meeting.

The surgeon did all the talking. He told them that he was sorry about the way things had turned out. He reassured them that the operation had gone perfectly from a technical perspective, and that he was both surprised and disappointed about the stroke.

He asked them to be positive as 'things often turn out better than they seem' and that 'people adapt to these things'.

Ben's wife explained how badly he had reacted to the smaller stroke and how certain she was that he would 'totally and utterly' hate being incapacitated in a nursing home. She said that they had no doubt that Ben would never want things done to try to save him for such a future; he would rather die.

The surgeon suggested that they had a duty to 'try'. He went further, suggesting that if they loved Ben they would want to 'do their best' for him and wouldn't want to 'just let him die'. He suggested that it would 'just be routine' to do the tracheostomy; he implied that it was 'part of ordinary care'.

It was very awkward to watch, but the family weren't deterred.

Ben's daughter was first to respond. She told the surgeon that they would never consent, because it would be 'exactly what Dad wouldn't want'. They appreciated the surgeon trying to do the operation, and didn't blame him for the outcome. They saw it as a gamble that everyone had accepted — but as a gamble that had been lost.

This family clearly saw the decision as their responsibility, and they were not going to consent. They were clearly sorry to upset the surgeon, but they weren't going to let his view influence them. They observed that he seemed to be 'living on a different planet'. I felt this rather nicely described the gulf between them.

The surgeon threatened to take his demand for consent to court. United, mum and daughter stared him down, daring him, confident that their firm, shared interpretation of Ben's interest would prevail. The surgeon gave in.

Neither a tracheostomy nor PEG were done — neither were ever mentioned again.

Ben died a week later.

Studies show that doctors are very hesitant to raise the possibility of limiting treatment with patients or families. This is a fraught area for doctors, because any mention of limits is easily misconstrued to suggest that the doctor 'wants to give up', 'doesn't care', or 'doesn't even want to try'. It is easy to see why doctors would want to avoid this.

Doctors want the possibility of limits to be raised by patients (or family) — but patients and families want the doctor to bring it up. As both wait for the other to 'break the ice', it never gets discussed — so unwanted, ineffective treatment just happens.

Most doctors respond well when patients or family members *do* bring up the subject. Raising the topic of 'how far to go' seems to be an important step for patients and family members to take. The sorts of questions that invite discussion include, 'We are very worried about where all this might end up. Can we talk about it?' or 'Can we talk about exactly what this treatment means for him?'

Sometimes the doctor's response can be reticent, with a response such as 'We can talk about that later — let's be hopeful now.' In this case, a more forceful request may be required, along the lines of 'No. We are concerned that we have come to a crossroads, and I think we really need to understand so we can make the right choice now.'

It is important to tell doctors that it is OK to give a frank, balanced, and honest assessment (otherwise there is a tendency to exclusively focus on hope). Here are a few suggestions that can work well:

'Please can you tell me as honestly as you can what is ahead? I really want to know so I can plan.'

'Without being overly optimistic, can you explain what I should expect?'

'What do you really think is the most likely outcome?'

'Can you outline the risks of each choice for us?'

These sorts of questions are tough to ask, because the answers can often be confronting — but they are important, because they give the doctor clear permission to reveal facts.

It is also important to be able to ask for advice. This is an entirely reasonable and sensible thing to do, especially as the medical issues are often very complex and rather uncertain. It asks a knowledgeable doctor to combine medical knowledge with their own humanity, and to think about what they might choose in similar circumstances.

'What do you advise?'

'What would you do in my situation?'

Knowing what the doctor would choose (or suggest) often provides really useful information to assist decision-making. Of course, there is no obligation for any patient (or family) to do what the doctor would do — it's just one more thing to throw into the mix.

Although it seems sensible to ask advice, some doctors will never give it (particularly about life-and-death choices). They suggest that everyone is different, and that these differences have such an influence on decision-making that they can't advise.

So even though the request for advice may get an unhelpful answer, or no answer at all, it still seems worth trying. And it can always lead on to more questions to understand why the doctor is advocating a particular approach, and whether his (or her) reasons resonate with your priorities. It is always important to take any advice with caution. Doctors may have such biases that their opinion may be virtually worthless (one study showed that the most influential factor causing doctors to recommend a controversial treatment was the availability of the treatment in their hospital).

It is also important to consider (and learn to recognise) medical dominance — there are numerous ways that those in the medical system can use power to coerce.

Often, patients will be lying in bed while the family will be sitting. In this situation, doctors often stand over sick patients (and families) when talking. This creates a submissive situation for the patient and family. By standing, the doctor also conveys a message that this will be a short meeting addressing the doctor's agenda (to 'tell' rather than to 'listen').

Asking for a 'proper, sit-down meeting' is advisable — especially where the issues are sensitive, complex, and important. Medical dominance does not support the shared, balanced roles that we believe to be important for effective interactions and good decision-making. It is important for patients and families to recognise dominant medical behaviour and to request a more appropriate communication.

Families often ask that 'everything' be done.

To doctors, 'everything' means every possible treatment that medicine can deliver — however unpleasant and however unlikely it is to work. Such a plan is generally misguided.

In many cases, it's because doctors ask the question, 'Do you want us to do everything?', which dictates this response from the family.

Families often interpret the question as 'Do you want us to do our best?' (of course we all want to do our best for someone we love) or worse, as 'Do you want us to try at all?' (where 'not even trying' would seem pathetic and wrong).

Asked in this way, almost all families feel compelled to demand everything.

It's incredibly difficult for a family to agree to do less than everything possible to save a loved relative — someone for whom they 'would do anything'. Love means doing everything, and doing less suggests that we don't love.

Because the effect is so predictable, we try to dissuade doctors from asking families if they want 'everything' — but you may still be asked. You need to be prepared to protect against a reflex response. You would be well advised to reformat the question in your mind to imagine the doctor is asking, 'Is there any limit to the awfulness of the treatments we can give or the minuteness of the chance of success we should strive for?' Thinking like this should help you to more clearly consider the issues and to answer appropriately.

Another thing doctors do is to present choices as a request to 'consent to treatment' in a way that makes it seem expected or reasonable to agree. Examples of this sort of approach include the following sort of comment:

'We need to operate.'

'He has to go to hospital.'

'We just need you to consent.'

In many cases, what the doctor is suggesting may turn out to be what ends up being agreed — but there is almost always an alternative that should be mentioned and considered (e.g., *not* having surgery, or *not* going to hospital and instead staying at home).

Awareness of all the options and open consideration of the options are important prerequisites for good decision-making.

Patients (and families) frequently opt for high-risk surgery because it seems to offer a chance of getting better (however remote), while the worst outcome seems to be to die on the operating table (without ever waking up). It seems like there is nothing much to lose.

Unfortunately, for those taking this option, very few patients actually die on the operating table. Frail, failing, chronically ill (high-risk) patients now mostly die after operations after a long struggle in ICU, or on the general ward, failing to get over their operation, or during prolonged convalescence as they fail to get back to health and suffer repeated complications.

Clearly, these patients *do* have something important to lose — they lose the opportunity for a good death, and they trade it for the discomfort of major surgery together with an unpleasant and protracted death. It is an important consideration.

It can be very helpful to reflect on how the word 'if' influences how we think about our end.

We regularly say 'if I get worse', 'if you get sick again', 'if it were to happen again'.

'If' suggests that an outcome is rather unlikely and unlucky. We use the word 'if' to make bad things seem more remote and to suggest that they might not happen.

Of course, the truth is that we all fail eventually — it's unavoidable — and as we get sicker, complications and relapses become more frequent and more certain. It helps planning if we are able to think and talk 'when' — 'when this happens again', 'when she can't recognise family'. Simply using the word 'when' keeps focus on planning for something that will occur, rather than erroneously suggesting that it won't (ever) happen.

It is useful to be aware that doctors feel they need to be *absolutely* honest about the possibility of survival. Honesty is clearly a good thing, but it can be unhelpful when discussing very poor choices. In medicine, almost nothing is 100 per cent certain — so addressing the discussion from the perspective of 'is there *any* chance that this treatment could work?' must inevitably elicit a positive answer 'there is a chance' — even where the chance is a billion to one.

Whenever the doctor admits there is a chance then most families feel compelled to 'go for it'. This leads to demands for treatment that has minimal chance of success, but which has a very high chance of being miserable, and which results in a bad outcome.

All this can be avoided by asking if there is a *'reasonable chance'*. This enables a degree of balance to enter the discussion and gets away from the need for absolute certainty.

Most of us don't interpret numbers well when it comes to risk; words seem to work much better, more vividly conveying concepts of risk and benefit. It can be helpful to confirm chances with doctors using words rather than probabilities. Confirming that the chance of a good outcome is 'virtually impossible', or 'very unlikely', or even simply 'unlikely' will generally encourage doctors to be more frank.

Exclusively focusing the discussion on survival is also unwise, because we know that people also have other priorities that are often more important. Doctors often limit the discussion to talking about survival — preventing death is a very important performance indicator for doctors — so patients and families have an important role to extend the discussion to include consideration of the impact of decisions on dignity, independence, and avoiding suffering.

It can also be helpful to ask about what has happened to other patients with similar conditions. This takes the discussion away from the individual patient, which can make worrying information less confronting.

There are other advantages, too. Asking about the experiences of others invites the doctor to convey a range of experiences; it also adds authority to the opinion, because it shows how it is based on a range of experiences. If the doctor seems to be providing an overly positive picture, it may be wise to ask if all patients have done so well or if some did worse. It is good to get a range of likely outcomes, and especially important where the best outcome is not 'worth it'.

Perfection (making the one 'right' decision) is a difficult thing to aspire to. To any problem, there can only ever be one perfect solution. This means that every other solution must be wrong, or failing in some way. Seeking perfection in situations where there is significant uncertainty (as in difficult medical decisions) is very stressful, and will often prove impossible.

Seeking to find and agree on a 'reasonable' decision can be much easier. It involves identifying 'unreasonable' or bad options, rather than trying to look for a perfect answer. Rejecting unacceptable solutions is something that we find quite easy to do.

Finally, a point on language. It is common to hear people talking of 'limitation of care' or 'withdrawing care' in discussions about choices at the end of life. 'Care' seems to be the wrong word to use here. We should never wish to be 'careless' in our efforts, nor should we ever want to 'stop caring'. We don't cease to care, and (hopefully) this is not what is meant. It is always better to think of 'stopping unwanted or ineffective treatment'. We stop doing bad, ineffective things *because* we care.

Nurses often have closer and more prolonged contact with patients and families. This can provide valuable insights that others may miss. Nurses are highly trusted (surveys show that they are more trusted than doctors), and the nursing role is more clearly associated with 'care' than with 'cure'. This can lead to a clearer role as patient advocate.

Experienced nurses can often identify treatment decisions that seem to be based on the needs and priorities of the doctor, rather than the needs of the patient.

Clearly, nurses can be wrong (like everyone else), and any advice or information should be critically analysed and discussed — but they can often offer an important, additional perspective.

Kathy's story

Ruby had advanced breast cancer. Despite numerous courses of chemotherapy her disease continued to pop up everywhere and relentlessly progressed. She was back in hospital because of problems with the cancer in her spine and liver.

During the first night back in hospital, Ruby didn't sleep. She refused sleeping pills and wanted to talk. Kathy was the nurse on duty. The shift was quiet, and so she sat with Ruby for some time. Kathy was a good listener; she said little as Ruby talked.

She heard a lot about Ruby, her family, her disappointments, and her fears for the future. Ruby confided that she was accepting treatment only because she felt her oncologist would be upset if she didn't.

Over the next weeks, Ruby continued to deteriorate while her oncologist added increasingly toxic treatments. He talked of more experimental treatment.

Ruby became too confused to decide anything.

Eventually, Kathy spoke to the oncologist. He was unimpressed, and told Ruby that she should 'keep looking on the bright side'. He told her it looked like he might be able to get her into a new study.

Ruby had a wretched time over the next weeks. She died before any experimental drug arrived and the study drug was never mentioned again.

Ruby's family never spoke to Kathy.

Most nurses are comfortable talking with patients about dying, and most are very good at it. Patients easily talk to nurses.

When doctors raise the issue of death, it is always with the concern that this might be seen as failure or weakness — a sign that the doctor is 'giving up'. Nurses have no such constraint. End-of-life discussions with nurses are often more natural and more relaxed than those conducted by doctors. Patients describe talks with nursing staff as being more 'emotional' and 'human', while those with doctors are 'just about medical stuff'.

Nursing care is also not locked into an expectation of cure (doctors cure and nurses care). Often, the nurse will be there at the bedside when a sick patient wants to talk about the difficult things — frequently during those lonely hours in the middle of the night. Furthermore, a shared involvement with unmentionable, undignified things (that nurses manage so well) often provides a special trust and connection.

The ability of experienced nursing staff to get to know

patients' wishes and fears makes them an important advocate and a vital resource for families (and for wiser doctors).

It is important to ask the difficult questions, and in my experience, it's not too difficult. Most doctors will adapt when they are asked to do so — responding to questions is an important part of their professional role.

There are a number of questions that effectively get the information that is really necessary for informed decision-making regarding serious illness. They're difficult questions, but important ones:

1. What are the treatment options? Is there anything else?
2. What are the benefits and harms of each? How likely are they?
3. What are the chances of a full recovery? What happens otherwise?
4. Is there more information that you think I should have?
5. What does my future hold? What happens with this disease?
6. What will happen if I don't have this treatment?
7. What do you recommend? What would you do if you were me? Why?

Let's examine each of these questions to try to understand how each may help the process of decision-making:

What are the treatment options? Is there anything else?
This question expects all the possible options to be presented,

and signals that you don't want the doctor to select only his (or her) choice.

What are the benefits and harms of each? How likely are they?

This invites a risk-benefit assessment of each option. It encourages an impartial assessment of each option. This forces the focus well beyond the 'you need an operation' approach.

How do you rate my chances of a full recovery? What happens otherwise?

This is a very important two-part question, especially when full recovery is an important goal (as it often is). It establishes the chance of full recovery and identifies what the alternatives might look like.

Is there more information that you think I should know?

Good medical practice involves sharing all the 'material information' required by the patient to make a fully informed decision. This question makes it difficult for the doctor to unilaterally decide not to mention some options.

What does my future hold? What happens with this disease?

This invites honest explanation of the likely course of the disease; it identifies what is likely to happen. Knowing this is important, because these things inform the cost-benefit assessment.

What will happen if I don't have this treatment?

Decision-making depends on having full information. Understanding what *not* having treatment means is as important as understanding the implications of having the treatment. In serious illness, the implication of no life-saving treatment is often death. It is important that this is recognised.

What do you recommend? What would you do if you were me? Why?

This is a powerful question that can often be very revealing. Many doctors find it confronting. It asks them to combine the medical reality (of the disease and treatment) with a personal perspective, and specifically your priorities ('if you were me'). A thoughtful answer to this question can resolve the difficult task of balancing risks and benefits.

Asking 'why' provides a check to see which factor(s) the doctor has given most weight to in coming to a conclusion. It provides a check that the things that the doctor has considered are those that are important to you. There is no obligation to adopt the doctor's choice, but the process can be useful and illuminating — and it might be the right answer.

CHAPTER 7

Finally

I hope this book has helped to make something that we spend great effort avoiding thinking about into something that is interesting, thought provoking, and important.

Dying isn't something we can now do without thought; on the contrary, even a tiny bit of thought can make a lot of difference. Good care and good choices require thought. We decline to think at our peril.

I hope that an understanding of the things that influence our decision-making will ensure better choices and better treatment.

There are important actions for patients (and families) who want to avoid treatments that are unlikely to provide benefit, will add to suffering, and may simply prolong dying:

- Remember that your 'treating doctor', when it comes to the crunch, is generally not your own GP — it is more likely to be a hospital doctor whom you will have never met. You need to ensure that your wishes can be clearly communicated to this person (at a time when you probably won't be able to communicate at all).

- If you *do* want everything done to prevent you from dying, it is generally not necessary to specify this since doctors are 'programmed' to do 'everything possible'. But, to be safe, it is still wise to make your wishes clear if this *is* what you want, just in case they (or your family) think you don't want it.

- Carefully consider what you really do *not* want — this will be much more helpful (to others) than knowing what you do want or might want.

- It is best not to hedge your bets by suggesting that you might want a little bit of intensive intervention. Any suggestion that you 'could' want intensive medical treatment is likely to get you everything. It suggests you aren't sure (and 'not sure' gets you treatment).

- Be clear about both unpleasant treatment and poor outcome — would you want to reject both, or would you accept prolonged unpleasant treatment if you could eventually return to your current health?

- It is wise to formally appoint an agent to make

decisions on your behalf. This needs to be someone tough, who will represent you using the appropriate legal appointment applicable to your country, state, or territory (they are all a bit different) — this gives them lots of authority, which is good.

- Your decision-maker needs to be a good decision-maker, and someone who cares about you, understands you, and is able to make difficult decisions. They need to have a reasonably determined personality and not shy away from difficult situations. They need to be a good negotiator who has the ability to convince others (it's a tough job!).

- Spouses are often appointed, but they often have far too much emotional involvement to be ideal decision-makers.

- Make sure your decision-maker knows how much leeway you want them to have. Are they expected simply to ensure that a clear advance directive you have made is implemented? Or do you want them to make a decision based on an understanding of your wishes in *all* the circumstances of a future medical crisis?

- Be sure to tell any appointed decision-maker that you want them to make the final decision for you, and not to let themselves be overruled by forceful doctors or family.

- If the person you choose to be your decision-maker seems uncomfortable about taking on the role, then *don't force them* (they are likely to be hopeless which can often be worse than appointing no one). *Choose someone else* (remember that close friends outside the family can be good in this role).

- Ask your family to respect the person you have chosen to be your decision-maker and to respect the decisions they make — because this is your choice for your life. If you can, get them to promise. Appeal to love.

- Get a palliative-care referral early (if possible). Early referral opens the option to make palliation a priority if and when you decide that this is appropriate (and gives you the option of getting good palliative symptom control earlier than may be the case when it is left to doctors to refer you).

- Stick to your message about what you don't want and regularly reinforce it to everyone.

- Try to get your GP (who hopefully knows you and your condition) to advocate on your behalf to help you avoid things at the end of your life that you don't want. Get a letter of support for your plan from your doctor(s) (if possible).

Dying is a journey that we all must go on — the only uncertainty is when. Some of us will go on this journey soon, others will not go for a while, but go we must.

The journey can be rough.

I hope this book helps you to navigate your path (and the paths of those you love) and to avoid the pitfalls that so bedevil others.

Science says: 'We must live,' and seeks the means of prolonging, increasing, facilitating and amplifying life. Wisdom says: 'We must die,' and seeks how to make us die well.

—**Miguel de Unamuno,** 'Arbitrary Reflections'.

Resources

MyValues

myvalues.org.au

MyValues is a free online program where a set of specially constructed statements are presented that help you identify, consider, and communicate your wishes about how far you would want to go with medical treatment in the later stages of life. It constructs a profile that explains your values in relation to life, death, and medical intervention. Understanding your values will help your doctors and your family to make better choices about your medical treatment.

Dying to Talk

dyingtotalk.org.au

Dying to Talk encourages people of all ages and levels of health to talk about dying. Despite being something that touches everyone, death doesn't receive enough visibility. Dying to Talk aims to reach into the community to normalise dying and to help people work out what's right for them at the end of their lives.

The 'Dying to Talk Discussion Starter' guides you through talking with your loved ones.

Death over Dinner

deathoverdinner.org

Conversations about end-of-life care often take place at a hospital in the midst of a crisis. Many people die in a way they wouldn't choose, with loved ones left feeling guilty, bereaved, and anxious.

This program encourages people to organise a dinner with the express aim of getting people to talk about death — to, as they put it, 'participate in the most important dinner conversation we are not having'.

They provide a range of videos, reading, and support materials, as well as giving tips to get the conversation started. The party host chooses the guests and the menu, and then lets the wine and conversations flow. It's a nice approach.

Death Café

deathcafe.com

A Death Café is a discussion group, where there is a directed discussion of death with no predetermined agenda, objectives, or themes. The aim is to encourage thought without leading people to any conclusion or course of action.

Food again plays an important role — and cake may feature. It's another excellent idea.

NHS Choices

nhs.uk/Planners/end-of-life-care/Pages/planning-ahead.aspx

An advance care planning resource for those living in England, Wales, and Northern Ireland.

NHS Inform Scotland

nhsinform.scot/care-support-and-rights/palliative-care/
planning-for-the-future/make-an-anticipatory-care-plan

Information about anticipatory care planning for those living in Scotland.

Think Ahead

hospicefoundation.ie/programmes/public-awareness/think-ahead

Hospice-related advance care planning website for the Republic of Ireland.

'Speak Up'

advancecareplanning.ca

Extensive resources for Canadians interested in advance care planning.

Centres for Disease Control

cdc.gov/aging/advancecareplanning/index.htm

A comprehensive resource for residents of the USA who are interested in advance care planning.

National Institute on Aging

nia.nih.gov/health/advance-care-planning-healthcare-directives

An alternative resource for residents of the USA interested in advance care planning

'Five Wishes'

agingwithdignity.org/five-wishes

A simple process for advance care planning that is widely used in the USA.

Advance Care Planning Australia

advancecareplanning.org.au

This site provides information about advance care planning, including information about how legislation and forms differ across the different states and territories of Australia.